Indian Medicine Power

Other Brad Steiger books published by Para Research

Brad Steiger Predicts the Future
True Ghost Stories
Astral Projection
Kahuna Magic
Monsters Among Us

Indian
Medicine Power

Para Research
Distributed by Schiffer Publishing, Ltd.
West Chester, Pennsylvania 19380

Indian Medicine Power
by Brad Steiger

Library of Congress Catalog Card Number: 84-061049
International Standard Book Number: 0-914918-64-6

Printed by R. R. Donnelley & Sons Company
on 55-pound SRT II Paper
Edited by Marah Ren
Cover design by Ralph Poness and Bob Killam
Typeset by Camilla Ayers

Cover photo "Lodge of the Horn Society" from
Edward S. Curtis, *The North American Indian.*
Norwood, MA: Plimpton Press, 1928.
Vol. 18, page 192, reproduced by permission of
Tozzer Library, Harvard University.

Published by Para Research, Inc.
A division of Schiffer Publishing, Ltd.

This book may be purchased from the publisher.
Please include $2.00 postage.
Try your bookstore first.
Please send for free catalog to:
Para Books
Schiffer Publishing, Ltd.
1469 Morstein Road
West Chester, Pennsylvania 19380

Manufactured in the United States of America.
Third printing, May 1987, 8,000 copies
Total copies in print, 14,000

Contents

Introduction

In this age of time management, compartmentalized lives, emotions, and fears, it is refreshing to return to the natural ways in Brad Steiger's book, *Indian Medicine Power.*

He has captured the essence of Indian people and their cosmology. The basis of all Amerindian ritual is the creation of a reality that allows the individual to experience at-one-ment with self, group, and all of creation.

Steiger transports the reader from the present state of chaos to a reality of attunement to nature and self where relationships with all beings—two-legged, four-legged, creatures that creep, crawl or fly—is once again possible.

The relationship of the Medicine to the people is unique to the Native American. Faith and trust in the Medicine, the practitioner of the Medicine, and an acceptance of basic yet complex principles of multi-modality of realities and time/space relationships, keeps the Indian Medicine alive and gives it special relevance to our own time.

As a teacher of Native American Studies and an educational specialist in Cross Cultural Awareness, I recommend *Indian Medicine Power* to school administrators, librarians, social studies or history teachers, students, and tribal or village schools across the United States and in Canada, Finland, and the USSR.

Brad Steiger has demonstrated an uncommon insight into the sacred belief systems of the Amerindian. His reverence for the spirituality of the people makes reading and rereading this book a pleasure in the purest sense.

Indian Medicine Power provides each reader with a path from yesterday to tomorrow that allows for individual growth, awareness, and an accessibility to the ancient mysteries that continue to be practiced today.

Seekers of truth will experience spiritual enrichment as they travel through the pages of time with a people who understand balance and harmony. Brad Steiger has presented the story of The Medicine with integrity.

Donna Linstead
Seattle, Washington
October, 1983

1
Quetzalcoatl's Promise

According to legend, there once lived a wise and powerful prophet-king of the Toltec Indians of southern Mexico named Quetzalcoatl, the Feathered Serpent. Quetzalcoatl, often described as bearded and white or fair of skin, brought the Toltecs a spiritual philosophy of love and kindness, and he taught them to raise better crops, to advance their architectural programs and to fashion a rather sophisticated scientific structure. Quetzalcoatl shaped the Toltecs into the greatest nation in Mexico; and by the time the Toltecs were supplanted by the Aztecs, the Feathered Serpent had been elevated to the position where prophet became nearly indistinguishable from deity.

It is said that when Quetzalcoatl left the Toltecs to travel to a faraway place beyond their knowing, he provided them with a last prophecy.

He told his people that in time whitemen, who would resemble him only in appearance, not philosophy, would come from the eastern sea in great canoes with massive white wings. These whitemen would, in turn, be like birds with two kinds of talons. On one foot would be the gentle, soft talons of a dove; the other foot would bear the hard, powerful talons of an eagle. One set of talons would seek to hold the Indians in love and kindness, while the other set would be prepared to claw them and grip them fast in slavery.

A few hundred years after the arrival of these first whitemen, Quetzalcoatl promised, other whitemen would appear who would bear only the talons of the peaceful dove. At this time, Quetzalcoatl, or the spirit that was in him, would also return. The Indians would once again have pride in their ancestors, and they would earnestly seek to regain both the spirit and the wisdom of the ancient people. The Indians and the whitemen, who bore the feet of doves, would work together to build a new and better world of peace, love, and brotherhood.

The Aztecs, who inherited their culture from the Toltecs, corrupted the teachings of goodness bequeathed to them by Quetzalcoatl and introduced the dark and bloody elements of human sacrifice and the subjugation of other nations. When the Spaniards came from the eastern sea in their great canoes with the billowing sails that appeared to be massive white wings, Emperor Montezuma and his people delighted in what they suspected might be protracted intercourse with a race of men as wise and as kind as the great Quetzalcoatl. However, Cortez and his soldiers and priests soon revealed themselves as man-greedy rather than god-generous. In one hand the Spaniards held the cross of the gentle Jesus, but with the other hand their eagle's talons wielded the sword and touched off the cannon.

In desperation, Montezuma turned to the true teachings of Quetzalcoatl, but he was too late to assist his people in anything other than their destruction and enslavement. Mortally wounded by one of his own people, Montezuma was given a vision of the future, which he told to Tula, his favorite daughter.

Montezuma saw the Aztecs crushed and defeated. He saw the whiteman striding powerfully across the land, conquering and killing all who rose up against him. He saw the Indians suffering ages of wrong committed against them, but he also foresaw a day of splendor when they would once again become one of the deathless nations of the earth. This day would not occur, however, until there evolved a generation of men and women who respected sacred traditions and who understood correctly the concepts of God and freedom. With this understanding would come a new birth of compassion, in which the cross of the whiteman's religion would remain, but its priesthood would vanish.

In the book *Warriors of the Rainbow*, by William Willoya and Vinson Brown, a young Indian boy asks a wise old woman of the tribe why the Great Spirit permitted the whiteman to take away the Indian's lands. The old woman, remembering the words of the old wise ones, tells the lad why the whitemen were sent to the North American continent:

> . . . the white men come from a land where only white men lived, and it was necessary for them to come to this place where they would learn about other races and learn to live with them, and that one day, when the Indians got the old spirit back again, they would teach the white men how to really love one another and how to love all mankind. Now, because the Indians were humbled and made

> poor by the white man's conquest, they have been cleansed of all selfish pride. They are ready for a great awakening, and they will awaken others.

Has Quetzalcoatl's promise been fulfilled? Has his spirit returned to give the Amerindians pride in their ancestry so that they might once again demonstrate the power and the wisdom of the sacred traditions and lead us all to a new and better world of peace, love, and compassion?

Sun Bear, a Chippewa medicine man, who publishes *Many Smokes* magazine, told me: "This is happening now, because it is in harmony with our prophecies that foretold a time when there would be a return to our medicine and our ways on this continent.

"We feel that we are the traditional keepers and protectors of the Earth Mother, and we feel that there is coming a time when there is going to be a major cleansing and changing of things. At this time, according to our prophecies, there would be people returning to our philosophy and our direction.

"There are a lot of young people in the country today who are interested, and they are taking on the outer surfaces of Indian things, but they don't fully comprehend it yet. There are a great many of them who are going only part way in terms of our metaphysics, but they don't really understand the true significance of our philosophy, and they haven't really made a full commitment.

"One of the big problems with white youth, of course, is their whole cultural background. They grew up under a different type of culture, so that for many of them, getting into the Indian thing is like reading another book. They hover over it for a while, and maybe a bit of it hangs onto them, but they don't really make any full commitment.

"To the traditional Indian people, medicine is a life-long thing, and it has a really strong significance. To really appreciate and benefit from Indian medicine power, one has to have this conviction and feeling. You have to really be involved in it."

This involvement extends beyond putting on a headband, a beaded belt, and some moccasins.

[The author's questions appear in italics throughout.]

"Right," Sun Bear agreed emphatically. "A lot of people come to me and say that they want to learn about medicine power. They say they want to get into the spiritual thing. I tell them that the start of it is that they must first learn to walk on the earth with a good balance. That means you have to learn to relate to each other and to the Earth Mother and learn to live in real harmony with her.

"That's where the first problem comes in. Ever since the whiteman came to this country, he has operated on a basis that he wants to get to heaven, but he doesn't want to bother to take any real responsibility for the Earth Mother and for the things around her.

"If the whitemen can't find a balance and work in harmony with the land and each other and show real love here, we traditional Indians wonder what the Great Spirit would want with such a bunch of ding-a-lings. We feel that the first step is to learn to walk in balance on the Earth Mother, then seek the medicine power that comes with the Great Spirit."

The well-known actor Iron Eyes Cody admitted that he had to relearn many of the old traditions in order to be better prepared for the return of medicine power.

Iron Eyes: "I have always been a traditional man. I was a champion dancer, and I made easy money going around following powwows. I got into the movies as a technical director. In 1949, Cecil B. De Mille made an actor out of me in the Gary Cooper picture *The Unconquered.*

"I am fifty-six years old, and I and a lot of other people had got away from the old traditions. But then about eight years ago, our young people wanted to learn the old ways. We older Indians began to think then that the circle is going to come back. Our dream is coming true. We are all going to get back in the Great Circle of Life.

"I went into scouting work to teach the Indian boys to dance and sing—they even won merit badges, besides! The boys got merit badges, but the singing and dancing was taking me back to my tradition. I went right back into the old ways."

So you, like so many Native Americans, had to relearn many of the old ways that had nearly become lost to you.

Iron Eyes: "That is right. Many of us have forgotten our own Indian traditions. We say, 'Oh, well, now I am a Catholic. Why should I join the Native American Church?'

"I have come to the point where I have faith in all churches. I have a son who was an altar boy at a Catholic church. He was so devout, he even taught Latin to younger boys. Today he is living on the Ute reservation, working with a medicine man. That doesn't mean he is going to give up Christianity altogether, because he believes in all religion the way I do. I won't criticize anyone else, but I believe that now we've got to go with our Indian beliefs, our ways, and we must stick together.

"I was in one Sun Dance where a young boy of about eight or nine was participating in his first big dance. I was the Receiver of the Pipe, who brings in the pipe, the altar, and the skulls.

"This little boy's grandfather is a medicine man, but at his age, the boy was not pierced like the other dancers. Instead, they tied a rope around his shoulder. He pulled with the rest of the men, who were trying to break the flesh around the skewers in their chests and the rope attached to the Sun Dance pole. I know that little boy will one day be a medicine man.

"My son is a traditional Indian. He sings the Sun Dance song while I serve as the Receiver of the Pipe. I also sing with the Sun Dance singer. A Sioux by the name of Jackson Tail is the lead drummer. Eagle Feather is the conductor of the Sun Dance. He is a spiritual man, a medicine man, a Yuwipi man.

"I belong to the Yuwipi. We pray to heal people. We go into the sweat lodge to pray. Then, we go into a building, and in one hour of light, we go through all kinds of ceremonials and put the altar up and pray to the tobacco sacks and pray for the people who are there. After one hour, the light goes out, and the room is in total darkness.

"In the darkness, the medicine man, whom I myself have tied up, wrapped him with rawhide, lies before the altar. When the light comes on, the altar of a hundred and fifty sacks of tobacco tied by women are all rolled up. Nobody has moved. I know that nobody moved in the dark, because my son and I were singing in the darkness by the altar; and we didn't feel anybody go up in that area. So we have what you would call a spiritual happening!

"Our younger generation is picking up the old traditions, learning the languages, learning the songs, learning the mysteries of the Great Spirit.

"Right here in Los Angeles, we have about sixty thousand Indians. For many years I was on the Board of Directors of the Indian Center. I was forced to resign because I had to go to Spain to make a movie. But my point is that we have as much tradition right here in this city as you will find on several reservations, because we old-timers believe in teaching our children the languages, the songs, and the Indian way.

"I taught my sons my language songs, and my wife taught them her songs. My older boy is the champion fast-Oklahoma-style dancer. Here in Los Angeles, we have an Indian get-together where we sing and do the tribal dances every Saturday night.

"We must all please the Great Spirit. We must go back to protecting this country like we did once before—all of us, not just the Indians! We must not destroy; for when we start destroying our environment, we begin to destroy ourselves. What we have in our medicine is strong, you know that, and our medicine does a lot of things.

"We must please the Great Spirit!"

Don Wanatee is proud of his Mesquakie people because he feels that they have pleased the Great Spirit by remaining as true to the old traditions as possible while living near Tama, Iowa, the very center of the midwest Bible Belt.

Don Wanatee: "I think that at least 70 percent of all Indians living today have lost their basic beliefs, but I believe that most of them want to go back to the old ways. The trouble is, they have had no ways or means of going back. We believe once an Indian loses touch with the old way, he can regain it, but he must be shown the way.

"There are a few pockets of Indians throughout the country that have maintained basically the same type of religion that their tribes have practiced for hundred of years. The Mesquakie is one of these people who have held on to their old ways.

"Of course, we have had many inroads of conversionary types of religion, including Indians from the West, some from the North, who contributed the peyote and drum societies, which are held in high esteem by some of the Mesquakie because they reflect some of the old religious ways of their forefathers. The Native American Peyote Church, of course, combines the old ways with Christianity, and the Drum Society combines with a Chippewa belief, to which some of the Objibwa up north in Minnesota still adhere. To expect things to be exactly as they were three hundred years ago is not realistic. The Mesquakie have changed their methods of practicing their beliefs; but, the basic ingredients of those beliefs remain the same as they were four or five hundred years ago. That is why I tend to believe them."

So you have always been a traditionalist?

Wanatee: "Yes. There have been times, especially in my younger days in grade school, that the missionaries of the Presbyterian Mission used to ride out to the settlement and try to convert us. They taught us verses and hymns, and told us how bad our religion was and how good theirs was. I have had moments like those, but they have reaffirmed my belief in the Mesquakie way."

Indian metaphysics are spreading out from those traditional practitioners of the old ways to affect our entire nation. Do you think there is a reason for this to be happening now?

Wanatee: "Yes. I think it is happening because this land itself is Indian, and the ancestors of the many tribes are still on this earth, only in a different state. The Mesquakie believe that the thin veil between life and death is so slim that the dead may influence the living.

"In my estimation, the younger generation perceives the faults and the incongruities of Christianity, which is supposed to be one of the better of the great religions of the world. Some of the practices and shenanigans that go on by professed Christians are not the Indian way. The Indian way is that you maintain your religious beliefs as part of the life that comes to you from the earth. Life comes from the earth. You don't give earth its life; it gives life to you. I think the Indian can show the younger generation—whether they be white or black or whatever—the proper way of treating life. Life is not a commodity. Life is a process.

"What non-Indian people need to do is to look at themselves and then develop a basic philosophy that will enable them to come into an understanding of what the earth holds for them. They should create a new religion. Some of their old religion is good, too; but, remember it came from the Old Country.

"The young people are beginning to understand. I can see it in their life-styles. I remember about twenty years ago, great white America was making fun of the Indian because of his dress style, the cut of his hair, the color of his skin, the way he lived in old huts, shacks, and tents—everything about the Indian was put down. But now I see many of the young people living that same way, and nobody really cares, because most of the predominant society—I did not say the dominant society, but the *predominant* society—think they are a lost cause, much the same as they thought the Indian was a lost cause fifty years ago. The younger generation is accepting more and more of the Indian ways."

I asked Dr. Walter Houston Clark, professor emeritus of Andover Newton Theological Seminary, to respond to the question of why we might be witnessing a return of the spirit of Indian medicine at this time.

"I think our civilization has overemphasized the rational faculties of man," Dr. Clark said. "Our ideas of science have been so restrictive that the essential nature of human beings is being starved. Unconsciously, modern man is reaching out for something that goes beyond the purely rational, the purely scientific. Our young people are ready for an expression of the intuitive side of their natures. The psychedelic drugs have been perhaps as important a catalyst as any in disclosing to these young people their essential natures, and I am sure that this is one of the reasons for the amazing concern about meditation and religion of many kinds among the young people.

"In the American Indian, our youth find a person who has expressed a simpler kind of existence that coincides with their desire to get away from the cities and to associate themselves with nature in order to live a life sufficiently simple in its essential needs so that there is a little more time for thought and consideration of what it is that makes life worthwhile."

Twylah Nitsch, a granddaughter of the last great Seneca medicine man, observed that whenever she attended an Indian get-together, she noticed a spiritual aura connected with each Indian present. "It is always there whenever we are together," she said. "You don't even have to mention it, for it is there."

"The rebirth of Indian medicine power will also bring with it an emphasis on *humanhood,*" Dallas Chief Eagle, a Sioux and the author of *Winter Count,* told me. "I must tell you a little story about how, back in 1947, I came to have a better understanding of the two major rules of life.

"I had returned from the marines, and I used to visit an old-timer to bring him a piece of roast, coffee, and bread so he would sit and talk with me in Indian. I could imagine that during his long lifetime, ministers and all kinds of missionaries had come to visit him. I used to tell him what I had observed in the outside world and tell him about the things I read.

"Once we got on the subject of religion, and I said, 'Grandpa (we refer to all our elders in the tribe as grandfather and grandmother), the whitemen have Ten Commandments to serve as their major guideline in life. Do we, as Indians, have any major rules or commands in life?'

"The old man said, 'Grandson, we have only two: First we love the Great Spirit and we always pay homage to Him. Second, we love *humanhood* (you cannot even find the word humanhood in the whiteman's dictionary). And I think, grandson, this is why we lost the country, because we were believers in humanhood and in these two major rules of life.

" 'But the Great Spirit is everything and everywhere, and because he is everything, he is also a humorist. He likes to laugh. I'll bet he laughs every day because he gave the whiteman eight more rules to confuse him!' "

I have long observed that mystics always get along famously, regardless of their ancestral or cultural backgrounds. Dogmatic differences in religions mean nothing to them, because they operate in a spiritual sphere that concerns itself with the dynamics of the cosmos, rather than the details of ecclesiasticisms. In the course of gathering material for this book, I asked a number of psychic sensitives for their impressions regarding American Indian mysticism and the resurrection of the Great Spirit.

Irene Hughes, the internationally known seeress of Chicago, is one-quarter Cherokee, and she has many fond memories of her maternal grandmother's wisdom and of her knowledge of herbs and healing. "Grandmother wasn't very tall, but she was slender and she had very dark hair and very black eyes. She was a woman of deep perception," Irene recalled as she reflected on her childhood in Tennessee.

"There is a tremendous interest growing in our Indian heritage," she continued. "I feel that the government will take a greater interest in the rights of the Indian and assist in preserving some of the benefits that come from their wisdom."

Do you think that the fact that you were able to discuss openly your dreams and visions as a child may have been due to your mother's acceptance of her own mother's ability to use her dreams to guide her life?

Irene Hughes: "Yes, I think my family had a greater tolerance of my abilities because of our Indian heritage. 'Knowing' could be regarded as a natural way of life."

I recall that many times you have mentioned that you were never made to feel odd or peculiar when you told your father to get the crop harvested in a hurry because a storm was on its way.

Mrs. Hughes: "That is true. I was absolutely never made to feel odd. My predictions were followed as a natural way of life."

Do you see any special insights that our American Indian heritage may offer us today?

Mrs. Hughes: "I feel that one of the very distinctive things is going to be the intense interest in herbs that Indians use and the medicinal advantages of them.

"I feel that we are truly evolving to a higher spiritual vibration. I feel that even the marijuana that our young people have been smoking may somehow be aligned with some of the hallucinogenic substances which some of the ancient people smoked in order to place themselves into an altered state of consciousness. Unfortunately, too many of our youth have prostituted the use of marijuana, and I feel much better about their going into meditation. It is wonderful that kids today are taking the time to meditate and to tune in.

"The fight against pollution is yet another way by which we may reach the Spirit of God. Indeed, we are having an evolution of spiritual growth in many different ways.

"I see that small groups will replace the organized church and that these powerful little groups will be filled with the Holy Spirit and with divine fire. I see that we will go into different types of rituals and develop once again a worshipful attitude toward nature.

"I feel that we will take a step higher in our spiritual evolution when we begin to realize that some of the ancient teachings were far better than so much of our modern philosophy. I see that we will perhaps go even deeper into those ancient teachings with a new understanding."

Those metaphysicians who believe that an acceptance of the doctrine of reincarnation can provide us with answers to many otherwise imponderable questions have stated that many of the slaughtered Indians, who were killed before their time by the encroaching whites, are being reborn today as white youth. This is the reason, these metaphysicians say, that coincident with the restoration of Indian magic, we are witnessing large numbers of young white people affecting both the manner of dress and the life-style of the American Indian. I asked those I interviewed to respond to the question of reincarnation and karma in regard to the resurrection of the Great Spirit:

Don Wanatee: "I do not believe that our ancestors could be reborn as whites, but I think there is that possibility among the Indians. Some of us probably have gone to the other side and have come back again in the form of another person, yet we are still in the same tribe. But as far as the white children are concerned—no, I cannot believe it. If they find a way to communicate with their own ancestors, I imagine they could come up with a new type of religion whereby they might be able to do it, but it would be difficult."

Don Wilkerson, director of the Arizona Indian Centers in Phoenix: "I tend to think that there is a strong possibility this may be happening, but I don't know. I don't fight the unknown; I accept it. I don't personally believe in that form of reincarnation, although my people [Creek-Cherokee] have a form of reincarnation and so do many other tribes. I won't deny that there are some strong elements of proof in the world that reincarnation exists. Whether it happens to us or not, I don't know. I do know that in some tribes belief in reincarnation is so strong that they will even point to someone and say that he was living before and say who he was."

Deon, psychic sensitive in Chicago: "Rather than reincarnation, this phenomenon seems to me to be more of an evolutionary thing. I think the children of today are more in tune with the universe, and they are reverting to a more simple lifestyle. The vibratory forces of the Indian, Indian awareness, may be influencing them without their knowing it. Now it is possible that this awareness may come from a past life, but it could also be due to the fact that someone in spirit with an Indian background may be guiding them. These young people want to live close to the earth; they want to grow their own things; they want to eat right; they want to be where the air is clean and pure. They are searching, yet being led, by an inner awareness of spiritual customs of which the great majority of people are not aware."

Do you feel this Indian awareness could be an example of the dead influencing the living?

Deon: "At present, this awareness is emanating from an unknown quantity, but it is an inner awareness, a feeling, to which we are now closer than we have ever been. Even in the crowded city of Chicago, you can begin to feel the vibrations changing. You can even feel it in your bodies. It is as if a vibratory force is attempting to raise us higher spiritually so that we might attune ourselves to hear the cosmic forces. Many people are receiving these vibrations and interpreting them as feelings of nervousness. They feel as if they are out of place, and they can't quite keep their minds on things that are happening in the material world. I think someone is really trying to get through to us and make us more aware. I am sure there are many entities watching over us at this time."

It did not occur to me to ask Tom Laughlin if he felt that he might have lived a previous life as an Indian, but in his film *Billy Jack*, the actor-writer-director has provided the moviegoer with the unforgettable study of a half-breed Vietnam veteran who drops out of white culture in order to study ancient Indian lore.

The modestly budgeted film has become a counterculture classic of the young mystic-warrior who leaves his seclusion only to protect the students at an interracial Freedom School. *Billy Jack* won the Grand Prize at the Festival of the Nations in Taormina, Sicily (1971), as well as Best Screenplay ("Frank and Teresa Christina" are really Tom and his wife, actress Delores Taylor), and an NAACP Image Award.

When I interviewed Laughlin, I found him to be not only a very aware exponent of Native American medicine, but an individual who had learned the validity of its power through firsthand experience.

Tom Laughlin: "I believe very strongly in dreams, and I do think the dream is telling me something about myself I don't already know. If

I knew, I wouldn't need the dream to help me understand. I also know that it takes me sometimes as much as a year or two after a dream before I fully understand it."

What was the reaction of the Native Americans to Billy Jack, *Tom?*

Laughlin: "Let me put it this way. There were an awful lot of Native Americans who descended upon us in the making of the picture. Some of them had had dreams and things of that nature which they felt should be in the film. We have had Native Americans come to us since the picture and ask us to do some rather heavy things. They meet with us in our home, and we are involved in a lot of work that they are doing. These are some very powerful medicine-type people.

"One guy who is very heavy in this field brought a group of Native Americans who were more militant than mystical, and they told me that they did not like the Black Power-type salute at the end of the picture. Then about a month later they were arrested in Los Angeles. As they were being taken away in paddy wagons, all of the same guys, who were upset about that salute, put their fists up in the air. They sent me a picture of it afterwards and said, 'I don't know who your inspiration was, but you knew something we didn't know!'

"The reaction, by and large, has been very strong from the Native Americans and from medicine people. Rolling Thunder, the Shoshone medicine man, said that he considered it the first true Indian movie ever made. But we do have our detractors as well."

I was very impressed with the manner in which you presented Billy Jack's use of clairvoyance throughout the film.

Laughlin: "I wouldn't intellectualize it, but certainly I think we indicate that Billy has a way of knowing that goes beyond what we are used to at this time. I think the Indian is in tune with what we might call the unobstructed universe. I think Billy Jack is clearly in touch with some source of communication that most of us don't know about."

What inspired you to submit to that dramatic rattlesnake ceremony?

Laughlin: "Again, that was the Shoshone medicine man Rolling Thunder, who is a very big force in both the Native American political and religious movements. He came to us and said that he had been told that we were supposed to have that ceremony in the picture. He told me about it, and he went through it. He had previously taken some apprentices through it, but, to my knowledge, no whiteman had ever seen that ceremony before.

"Indians and people I trust told me that Rolling Thunder can walk down a road in the Nevada desert, walk a quarter of a mile inland, and there, under a rock, will be a rattlesnake. Rolling Thunder will talk to the snake, then come back on the road and go on his way.

"Rolling Thunder not only told us to put the ceremony in the movie, which we had not intended to do until he appeared, but he remained there throughout the entire filming. The morning we shot the scene, we went through a special ceremony. Rolling Thunder was there with a seven-foot rattlesnake, I wouldn't have submitted to the ceremony without Rolling Thunder being there."

[*From a studio press release:* "Since no known white men have been introduced to the snake ceremony, Laughlin's indoctrination was in itself deemed a precedent. Rolling Thunder, impressed with the star's sympathetic understanding of the mystical ways of the red man, explained: 'Being an Indian is not a matter of blood; it is a way of life.'

["In the actual ceremony, the candidate, after thorough purification and preparation, goes high on a mountain top and permits himself to be bitten over and over by a rattlesnake. According to the Indian, if the candidate has power and has been properly prepared, he will recover, absorbing the mana of the snake and thus become a 'brother to the snake.' Shoshone . . . means snake . . . .

[" 'The relationship between man and reptile in the Indian belief is highly spiritual, very personal and not transferable.' Thus even Rolling Thunder could not command the snake in the way that a trainer controls a dog. The only help Laughlin had was a helicopter which was an hour's flight from Santa Fe.

["While crew and cast marvelled at Laughlin's courage, Rolling Thunder was not surprised: 'It's why he's playing Billy Jack,' he said. 'In his heart he is Indian.' "]

Tom, I'm certain you've noticed that we are now witnessing a resurgence of Native American magic and mysticism.

Laughlin: "Yes, I think the drug movement was a colossal movement into the spiritual realm. The kids knew that there was something more inside of themselves than they had been led to believe. All of a sudden they realized they had a soul, and that there were things in the soul beyond a little ego structure. There were powers that could be stirred up—both good and bad—and experienced.

"The unfortunate problem with the standard religions in America is that they don't believe in the soul anymore. Orthodox religion has become an ego trip. You identify your ego with Christ, and you have that kind of super power. It doesn't seem to occur to them that there is really a mystical, transcendental experience inside everyone.

"So, I think that is what the drug thing was about. I think that is what the Maharishi was about. And as you know, the Maharishi came into power only because the Hopi closed their gates to the kids. The moment the Hopi reopened them a year later, the Maharishi came over and his tour fell absolutely flat.

"Brad, you know better than I that when the Indian approaches the drug, the peyote, or whatever, they really prepare and they know that God is there. They know that if they don't prepare, they can be taken away.

"The kids are beginning to realize that there is something more than a kick in drugs. They are gravitating toward the Indian, who has, in my opinion, kept this country together with his spiritual life.

"I think the center of the religious power structure is Taos Pueblo, which is the one place you can't find out their secrets no matter who you are. I believe it is because if they let their secrets out and that religious grace that is being held there were dissipated, our country would go totally down.

"We had Andy Vidovitch, Wovoka's [the Paiute Peace Messiah, originator of the Ghost Dance] spiritual heir, on location. Vidovitch is a very spiritual person. His wife, who is Wovoka's daughter, and his son had died a couple of years ago. Just before we started making *Billy Jack,* Andy was preparing to die. A water heater had blown up and had burned 80 percent of his body. He was lying there, wanting to go, when his wife appeared and sat on the bed and told him he couldn't die and permit Wovoka's message to die with him. He had to stay alive until we got the Ghost Dance part in the movie.

"But Andy wouldn't help me write the speech for that Ghost Dance scene. Every day he kept telling me not to worry about it. Finally it was time to shoot it, and he still wouldn't help me write it—so I wouldn't shoot it.

"The last day, I had to shoot something, and Andy said, 'You just go in there and that little fellow, that Holy Spirit, he will tell you what to say.'

"I went in there, and it was the most embarrassing time of my life. Honest to God, until I got back and saw the rushes, I had no idea what the hell came out of my mouth."

In other words, it was a spontaneous possession.

Laughlin: "Totally. Before I saw the rushes, I told Andy that we would have to leave the scene out of the movie. I told him that I couldn't think of a thing to say.

"He smiled, and said that I would love the scene. 'Wovoka spoke,' he said. 'You didn't speak.'

"I was amazed when I saw the rushes. There was a speech about how the spiritual life in America had failed the kids and how they had gone to drugs and that now they are looking for something more substantial. I was very stunned to hear all that.

"If Andy Vidovitch, Wovoka's son-in-law, had not been there when we did the Ghost Dance, there would have been heavy trouble. The Taos Indians were shocked to see that we knew the dance correctly. It has always been taken as a circle dance, which is totally different from the way we did it—not totally, but there are a couple fundamental things that make it quite a different dance from the spiritual point of view.

"If you go back and see the picture, you will see a man in khaki pants and khaki shirt and a hat standing outside the old *kiva* that we're in. That is Andy Vidovitch. I did not want him out of the picture. I wanted everything right. I didn't want to fool with that dance.

"I went into trance during that scene. I have a rule when I'm acting that no one else can say cut, because maybe I am going to go back and start the scene over, so no one can say cut. There are ten minutes of film in a camera's magazine. We started doing that dance, and when I finally said cut, I was shocked to find that twenty minutes had gone by. The camera had run out. Everyone was just standing there. No one dared to say cut.

"I thought it had only been a minute or two. The colors just got so incredibly beautiful, I got fascinated with them. After a while, I thought well, we've got enough film shot now; and I was stunned to find it was twenty minutes later. So if you did that dance properly all night long, I know what would happen!"

Tom Laughlin has tested the validity of Native American medicine for himself, and he has found that it does have a power and a relevance for the non-Indian. He has also learned that, as Rolling Thunder said, "Being an Indian is not a matter of blood; it is a way of life."

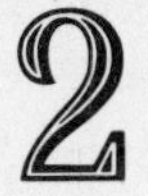

Medicine Power and the Cosmos

In an old book titled *The Fourteen Ioway Indians* (London, 1844), an account is given in which a packet ship was becalmed for several days near the English coast. A group of Native Americans were on board, and the captain decided to call upon their medicine man to "try the efficacy of his magical powers with the endeavor to raise the wind."

> After the usual ceremony of a mystery feast and various invocations to the spirit of the wind and ocean, both were conciliated by the sacrifice of many plugs of tobacco thrown into the sea; and in a little time the wind began to blow, the sails were filled, and the vessel soon wafted into port.

During the summer of 1865, the great warrior Roman Nose undertook many medicine fasts in order to receive protection from enemies. Under the tutelage of White Bull, an elderly Cheyenne medicine man, Roman Nose lay on a raft for four days in the midst of a medicine lake, partaking of neither food nor water, suffering a relentless sun by day and pouring rain by night. Spiritually equipped with the visions obtained during the fasts, and solemnly bearing the protective eagle-feather war bonnet that White Bull had fashioned for him, Roman Nose requested the honor of leading a charge against the Blue Coats who were invading the Powder River.

On the day of battle, Roman Nose mounted his white pony and called to the assembled warriors. He asked them not to fight that day for single honors, but to fight in a unit as the Blue Coats did. Then, to prove his medicine power, he told the warriors not to charge until he had ridden before the whites and caused them all to empty their guns.

Roman Nose broke away from the war party, urged his pony into a run toward the ranks of the white soldiers standing before their wagons. When he was near enough to see the Blue Coats' faces, he wheeled his mount and rode parallel to their ranks and their rifles.

Roman Nose had completed three or four passes before a ball from a Springfield musket smashed his pony from under him. Roman Nose rose, unscratched, and the massed Cheyenne and Sioux shouted their war cries and attacked the Blue Coats' lines.

In September 1867, Roman Nose was asked by the Sioux to join them in an attack against a group of white scouts, who had been sent by General Sheridan to search out Indian encampments for winter attacks. Roman Nose agreed to join the Cheyennes' allies; but first, he said he must undergo a purification ceremony. One of the women had inadvertently used an iron fork to prepare his food, and, since his medicine vision had told him that his power to turn away Blue Coat bullets would be destroyed if any metal contaminated his food, he must have time to restore his magic.

Although the Cheyennes respected their great warrior's wish, their impatient allies exerted pressure upon Roman Nose to abbreviate his purification rites. Roman Nose was not a chief, but he was the warrior-mystic who had inspired his people to continue to fight to protect their lands and their way of life. Courageous charges, brave deeds, and acts of honor would be sparked by Roman Nose's presence on the field.

Realizing that his medicine had been destroyed and that he would surely be killed that day, Roman Nose yielded to the Sioux's demands, painted his face, and placed his war bonnet on his head. He was cut down that day by Forsyth's Scouts in the fight the whitemen called "The Battle of Beecher's Island" and the redmen called "The Fight When Roman Nose Was Killed."

In the modern classic *Black Elk Speaks,* John G. Neihardt tells of accompanying the aged holy man of the Oglala Sioux to Harney Peak, the same place where the spirits had taken Black Elk in a vision when he had been young. The old man painted himself as he had seen himself in his great vision and called out to the Great Spirit to hear his prayer that the Indian people might once again find their way back into the sacred hoop, the Great Circle.

Neihardt writes that as those who stood by watched, thin clouds began to gather out of a clear sky. "A scant chill rain began to fall and there was low, muttering thunder without lightning. With tears running down

[his] cheeks, [Black Elk] raised his voice to a thin high wail, and chanted: 'In sorrow I am sending a feeble voice, O Six Powers of the World. Hear me in my sorrow, for I may never call again. O make my people live!' "

According to Neihardt, Black Elk stood for a few minutes in silence, his face uplifted, weeping in the rain. Soon, the sky was once again cloudless.

What makes American Indian medicine power work? How can sacred doctors summon wind, ward off bullets, squeeze rain out of cloudless skies?

Sun Bear, Chippewa medicine man: "Some people would think of these things as magic. We think of them as simply using forces that have been here for all time for our benefit or our needs. Magic is not 'magic' if you understand it. It is something that works. It is when you will something into existence because you have a need of it."

Rarihokwats, Mohawk, editor of *Akwesasne Notes:* "I'm not certain it is possible to respond to the question of what is the power evident in Amerindian magic. You see, the Power is the power of creation. Whatever that power is, it causes the grass to grow, the earth to rotate, and all the things that happen in all of creation. This is a tremendous power. It is the power to create life. And the more that Indian people or other people become acquainted with that power, the more they are able to internalize and utilize and flow with that power."

Is part of it the recognition that we are part of nature and everything is part of one whole?

Rarihokwats: "Yes, and the whole is contained in each part. It has to have both of those aspects. You are not only part of the whole, but the whole is part of you."

We are individuals, and at the same time, part of all. We are part of the cosmos, and the cosmos is part of us.

Rarihokwats: "Right, and in indistinguishable kinds of ways. If you just say, 'I am part of the universe,' then it is possible for you to withdraw from the universe at some point and set up your own separate shop. On the other hand, if the universe is part of you, and not only just a part that can be amputated, but a part upon which you are dependent, then you cannot separate yourself, you cannot withdraw."

Although we shall attempt to define the more subtle and sacred aspects of medicine power and the methods by which we might acquire those "indistinguishable kinds of ways" that will enable us to become one with the cosmos and acknowledge that the cosmos is one with us, we might be well advised to offer additional physical proofs of the efficacy of medicine power before we define the abstract elements inherent in American Indian magic.

Perhaps the best known demonstration of medicine power is the rain dance. The imagery of dancing Indians bedecked in colorful costumes, chanting prayers to the Great Spirit for life-giving moisture is firmly implanted in the white consciousness as the single most representative act of Native American magic.

There is no reason for the more knowledgeable students or practitioners of medicine power to be offended that such a ceremony has become stereotypical of a vast and serious cosmology. We are no less dependent upon the harvest of crops today than we were one hundred years ago. An adequate supply of food will never lose its impact as a basic issue in our survival as a species. There is not a farmer today so sophisticated that he or she has not wondered if the medicine of an Indian rain dance really works.

There seems little question that the ceremony, properly practiced, does most certainly provoke the fall of rain.

The northeastern section of the United States suffered its worst drought in recorded history when New York City was host to the World's Fair in the summer of 1965. As a promotion for the Niagara Falls' Maid of the Mist Festival in July and in order to alleviate the drought conditions, a seventy-five-year-old Tuscarora chief named Black Cloud performed a rainmaking ceremony on June 30.

Attired in full regalia, Black Cloud began the ritual at 10:25 A.M. Just a few moments before 11:00 A.M., raindrops began to splatter the fair grounds. Within an hour, Manhattan was experiencing what the weather bureau described as a "good rain shower."

Lorraine Carr, writing in the Albuquerque *Tribune* (June 5, 1972), states that the rain dances held at the Tesuque Indian Pueblo on May 28 brought a gentle five-hour rain that "soaked the thirsty mother earth."

Ms. Carr recalled the June day when she attended a dance at Santo Domingo Pueblo accompanied by two skeptical Texas friends. Although the blue sky was cloudless when they left Taos at 10:00 A.M., Ms. Carr brought her raincoat and umbrella. Her doubting friends were amused by her faith in the Indian's ability to produce rain.

> The Indians, dressed in their impressive regalia, danced rhythmically in the hot sun. They never missed a beat.

> About four in the afternoon the thunderheads had built up and here came the rain. I put on my raincoat and stretched my umbrella, while my friends and other spectators sought shelter.
>
> The rain came in torrents. As we started for Taos, we found the arroyos filled.
>
> As my host maneuvered the car through the swirling water he glanced at the sky still heavy with rain clouds and all he said was, "I'll be damned."
>
> I have attended many Indian dances for rain and the rains never fail to come. Someone asked, "Why not hire Indians to do rain dances rather than hire cloudseeders?"
>
> The Indians put little faith in such a rainmaker dance. It would anger the Great Spirit. The Indian has always been a partaker of nature, not a destroyer.

Snow, as well as rain, apparently can be "danced" into falling.

When Calgary Productions, a subsidiary of Walt Disney Studios, was filming the million-dollar movie *Nomads of the North* in 1959, the movie company found itself in an ideal location in the Kananaskis Forest near Banff, Alberta, Canada—ideal, except for the lack of snow. The ground was spotted with nothing more than a light film, and the seventy members of the company, together with one hundred extras, stood about waiting for snow to fall at a daily cost of thousands of dollars to Calgary Productions.

After five days of financial anguish, the moviemakers held a conference to discuss the problem. The use of artificial snow was rejected, because the cost of covering several acres would have been prohibitive. Then someone mentioned Chief Johnny Bearspaw and his Stony tribe, who had become well known for their successful rain dance at the Calgary Stampede.

Although Chief Bearspaw admitted that the Stony tribe had never before danced for snow, he saw no reason why it could not be done. He asked a fee of ten dollars per dancer, told thirty-two members of his tribe to turn out in full ceremonial costume, and the ceremony was performed.

Shortly after the dance had been concluded, seven inches of beautiful snow blanketed the Kananaskis Forest.

It would also seem that Native American medicine people have the ability to transfer this power to artifacts and religious icons.

On April 17, 1964, the new Anthropological Museum in Chapultepec Park in Mexico City installed a 167-ton statue of Tlaloc, Teotihuacan god of rain. The gigantic, twenty-four-foot idol had to be transported into Mexico City on a specially built trailer, and some of the streets en route had to be reinforced because of the statue's great weight. Carved from living rock about twelve centuries ago, Tlaloc had been found years before near Coalinchan, thirty-one miles east of Mexico City. When Tlaloc arrived in the Mexican capital, he was welcomed by a cloudburst that inundated the city and rained out ball games.

Some years ago, Professor William Payne, an archaeologist, ceramicist, and art professor, found a number of likenesses of the ancient rain god Cocijo while digging at the site of the ancient Zapotec civilization in Mexico. When Professor Payne returned to his classrooms at Orange Coast College in Costa Mesa, California, he produced several ceramic copies of Cocijo and decided to try an experiment. He selected a day when the skies were cloudless and the weather forecasters had decreed that no rain was in store for Costa Mesa, then he placed the icons about the campus and convinced his students to join him in a rain-making ceremony.

By 2:30 that afternoon, the college and the community were being drenched by rain.

Since that first experiment in 1953, Professor Payne and his students have produced rain on days when clear weather has been predicted, for a total of twelve hits out of thirteen attempts. For the skeptics who were stunned enough to see an academician and his students provoking rain out of formerly cloudless skies by conducting ceremonies involving icons the size of a man's palm, four of the rainstorms came in on southerly winds from Mexico, an occurrence which is uncommon in the Costa Mesa area.

"The correct placement of the effigies involves quite a bit of work," Professor Payne commented. "That's why I don't perform the ceremony more often. Then, too, I only like to do it when rain is really needed. I won't offer theorizations as to why these ceramic figurines produce rain, except to say that they do. After all, perhaps in a few thousand years, many of the things we do today will be considered strange by future civilizations."

On June 5, 1964, the citizens of Prosser, Washington, decided to throw convention to the wind and conduct a rain ceremony in an attempt to coax rain to fall on their parched community. At first the faithful produced only a slight drizzle, but then more than a thousand of their neighbors, encouraged by the initial success, joined the ritual with noisemakers. The drizzle that had been flecking the dry soil became a welcome downpour.

Yes, it seems entirely possible that professors, students, farmers, and townspeople can capture the essence of medicine power and utilize it to their advantage—if the need is great enough and if their belief is strong enough.

"I really believe the power of American Indian medicine comes from an attitude of acceptance," Don Wilkerson, director of the Arizona Indian Centers in Phoenix told me.

"The traditional Indian people understand that there is both good and evil and that these things can be influenced by our actions. If you develop an attitude of acceptance toward the unknown, you can make things happen. The Indian is not hung up with controlling nature, but he knows that he can guide it. And if he learns to understand it, he knows that he can live with nature and have it nurture him."

In July 1970, fifty farmers from Hanska, Minnesota, most of them of Scandinavian ancestry, gathered in Native American costumes to perform a rain dance. They formed a circle to beseech the heavens for moisture for their dying crops, and they sought to encourage spiritual intercession by conducting their supplication in a manner indigenous to the North American continent. Adding to the physical stimulus and giving evidence of their faith and optimism, two of the farmers wore raincoats over their costumes. Their dance was received, and a thunderstorm released two inches of rain on their parched farmland.

Was the performance of a rain dance ceremony an act of cultural regression on the part of the Minnesota farmers? Or do people all over the world of all ancestral strains conduct the same kind of reaching-out rituals in their times of greatest need? Do we not, wherever we may choose to dwell, have the same common spiritual ancestry, receive the same revelations from Higher Intelligence, and express ourselves in similar ritual acts, whose origins may be but dim memories in the collective unconscious?

In *The World's Rim,* Hartley Burr Alexander observes:

> . . . There is something that is universal in men's modes of thinking, such that, as they move onward in their courses, they repeat in kind if not in instance an identical experience—which, if it be of the mind, can be understood only as the instruction which a creative nature must everywhere give to a human endowment. The Indian gives us an understanding of life colored and adorned by his own unique familiarities with a hemisphere of Earth which for many centuries was his only; this understanding is delivered in his own imaginative

> guise and following the impulses of his own artistic genius. But the fact that so created—by a unique people in a unique continent—it still in substance echoes what other groups of men in other natural settings have found to be *the human* truth, so that Aryan and Dakota, Greek and Pawnee, build identical ritual patterns to express their separate discoveries of a single insight, is but the reasonable argument for a validity in that insight which cannot be lightly dismissed. . . .

While recognizing the American Indian's uniqueness, numerous metaphysicians have drawn comparisons between many tribal rituals which would certainly appear to be "echoes" of what "other groups of men in other natural settings have found to be *the human* truth." At the same time, it may be seen that due to their hundreds of years of isolation from both East and West, the American Indians may have preserved the essentials of the ancient mysteries in their purest form.

The traditional Indian makes medicine work, and the power of this magic is usually of a higher efficiency than that of the average student of Western occultism. These men and women who seek the power of medicine must make a more total commitment and pay a higher price in self-denial to attain the *wakan* (the essence of medicine) than is required of any initiate in the schools of European white magic.

To be a recipient of medicine power, the practitioner must live the commitment every moment of every day. The practitioner must believe in the unity and the cooperation of all forms of life, and must cherish and value all brothers and sisters.

When one must take the life of an animal in order to survive, the practitioner of medicine power kills only after uttering a prayer, as if performing a sacrament. The entity (the soul of the animal) and its group spirit must be told that such an act is necessary in the turning of the great wheel of life. It may well be that the traditional saying of "grace" before meals is an unconscious method of duplicating this propitiatory prayer.

The vision quest, certain meditative techniques, and innumerable symbols employed in a wide variety of American Indian ceremonies are reminiscent of Tibetan mysticism. Attending any powwow, especially those in the Southwest, one will be struck by the similarities between the masks, the headdresses, the boots, prayer wheel-like devices, and dozens of symbolic designs that are but variations on the classic Tibetan mandala. When one uses a mandala in meditation, one is to discover God in the center of the design, as He is in the center of the universe. The four parts that surround the "eye of the Great Spirit" represent the

Four Directions, the Four Seasons, the Four Ages of Man, the Four Kingdoms of Life; and as we shall learn, four is the number of power in Native American medicine.

Carl Jung once warned Westerners that they should be cautious of an extended practice of yoga, as it was not a metaphysical practice of the soil on which they had been reared. Although there are basic spiritual insights which are universal, there may be unique modes of attaining extended awareness, illumination, and cosmic consciousness that have been given to certain peoples and places to more effectively achieve communion with the Great Spirit within the confines of cosmically determined borders. If this is true, then the American Indian vision quest, during which the seeker goes into the wilderness alone to fast, to receive a spirit guide and a secret name, not only provides us with a prototype of the revelatory experience and the means of obtaining medicine power, but it may provide us with the peculiar mystical experience that is most efficacious for our hemisphere.

Hartley Burr Alexander saw the continued quest for wisdom of body and mind—the search for the "single essential force" at the core of every thought and deed—as the perpetually accumulating elements in medicine power. The reason the term "medicine" became applied to this life-career function is simply because those attaining stature as men and women, who had acquired this special kind of wisdom, were so very often great healers. The true meaning of "medicine," of course, extends beyond the arts of healing, clairvoyance, precognition, and the control of weather elements.

Medicine power enables its possessor to obtain personal contact with the invisible world of spirits and to pierce the sensory world of illusion which veils the great mystery. As the Eastern holy man intones his mantra and sings holy syllables in an effort to attune himself with the eternal sound, the cosmic vibration, so does the traditional Native American seek for magical songs which will increase the power of the medicine.

Alexander states the following in regard to the importance of the song in Native American medicine power (*The World's Rim*):

> One cannot too strongly emphasize the fact that for the red man the discourse of song is in itself a magical, or indeed a spiritual thing. His music is his most certain means of impressing his sense of need upon the Powers, and of bringing them into communion with himself. His singing is not at all primarily for his companions in

> the world of men, but for the spirit beings that envelop the human realm. Ceremonies are of greater efficacy if the songs are repeated at greater length. . . .

With his personal songs to reestablish his position with the mysteries about him, the traditional American Indian regards life as an ordeal during which he must continually prove himself and pursue his quest for wisdom of body and soul. Although certain religious traditions may vary from tribe to tribe, the central feature of medicine power is the reliance upon individual visions as the fundamental guiding force in the ordeal that is life upon the earth plane.

The generalities given above by way of definition of medicine power are valid, because the dogma of tribal rituals is always secondary to the guidance one receives from personal visions. The traditional American Indian cherishes individuality above all things, and guards personal sacred revelations with the utmost secrecy. Because of this emphasis upon individualism and the sacredness of personal visions, the world is far more familiar with the mysticism of nearly any other people than it is with the teachings of the American Indian.

It would seem a fair statement to make that the Native American has been far more interested in meditation than in communicating personal visions to others. Even the songs of revelation bear the indelible stamp of the individual soul, and that song cannot be sung by another until the creator has either given it or sold it.

In the same manner, tribal rituals came originally to an individual visionary who transmitted the song and the dance only to carefully approved initiates.

Hartley Burr Alexander writes, "Even in the great food-winning ceremonies, such as the game and corn dances, while these are cosmically timed and set by nature, nevertheless in their mythic backgrounds is invariably recognized some personal adventure or sacrifice: some seer adventuring the wilderness that he may bring thence the secret teachings of the gods that will lure forth the food-animals. . . the ritual is only the outer and incidental setting for the man's self-proof and inward vision. Throughout, the central conception is dualistic and dramatic; the natural world and the social provide the scene and the spectacle, but in the man's soul is the action."

John Collier sees the American Indian's "ancient, lost reverence and passion for human personality, joined with the ancient, lost reverence and passion for the earth and its web of life" as crucial elements which the world has lost, but must regain, lest our species die. In his *Indians of the Americas,* Collier states:

> This indivisible reverence and passion is what the American Indians almost universally had; and representative groups of them have it still.
>
> They had and have this power for living which our modern world has lost—as world-view and self-view, as tradition and institution, as practical philosophy dominating their societies and as an art supreme among all the arts.

As we have noted repeatedly, Indian medicine is fully cognizant of the nurturing Earth Mother, of one's total involvement in the web of life, and of one's inability to separate from the cosmic flow. Charles Alexander Eastman (Ohiyesa) observed in *The Soul of the Indian* how a nearness to nature kept one in touch with unseen powers:

> I know that our people possessed remarkable powers of concentration and abstraction, and I sometimes fancy that such nearness to nature . . . keeps the spirit sensitive to impressions not commonly felt, and in touch with the unseen powers.

William Willoya and Vinson Brown, authors of *Warriors of the Rainbow,* believe that there is a ". . . great strength in the earth and in nature that the old Indians knew about, but which is almost lost to present generations."

Willoya and Brown acknowledge the possibility that farmers who love the soil and that those who live in the wilderness for long periods of time may experience the mysterious feeling of a kinship with nature that enables one's "whole being to become sensitively attuned to both wild life and plants." However, they feel the ancient Indians were able to achieve an even greater sense of harmony with all life:

> The Indians . . . went a step beyond this to the point where the human spirit in some way, possibly never measurable by scientists, used the animal spirit as a tool in reaching the Source of the World and in purifying the soul. The great, pure-hearted chiefs of the olden times achieved their spiritual power by the most difficult self-discipline, fasting and prayer, including the utter emptying of the heart of all earthly desires and the tuning of the inner ear to the whispers of the wilderness. This was not idol worship . . . but something far deeper and more wonderful, the understanding of the Spirit of Being that manifests itself in all living things. . . .

In my opinion, another crucial element in the spiritual chemistry that comprises medicine power is the ability to rise above linear time. Our conventional concept of time, existing in some sort of sequential stream flowing along in one dimension, is totally inadequate to provide one with a full assessment of reality. This one-two-three kind of time may be convenient for us when we are in an ordinary, conscious, waking state, since it limits the input of sensory data and allows us to deal effectively with the "present"; however, I believe that our essential selves can rise to a level of consciousness wherein past, present, and future form an eternal now; and I believe that we may gain access to this level of consciousness in our dreams and visions.

In his text for Ira Moskowitz's book of drawings, *American Indian Ceremonial Dances,* John Collier comments upon the Indian's possession of a time sense that is different, and happier, than the whiteman's:

> . . . Once our white race had it, too, and then the mechanized world took it away from us . . . We think, now, that any other time than linear, chronological time is an escapist dream. The Indians tell us otherwise, and their message and demonstration addresses itself to one of our deepest distresses and most forlorn yearnings. . . .
>
> . . . Did there exist—as the Indians in their whole life affirm—a dimension of time—a reality of time—not linear, not clock-measured, clock-controlled, and clock-ended for us, we would be glad; we would enter it, and expand our being there. There are human groups, normal, and efficient in difficult ways of the world, which do thus expand their being, and the tribal Indians are among them.
>
> In solitary, mystical experience many of ourselves do enter another time dimension. But under the frown of clockwork time which claims the world, we place our experience out in an eternity beyond the years and beyond the stars. Not out there did the other time dimension originate, in racial history, but within the germ plasm and the organic rhythms and the social soul; nor is its reference only or mainly to the moveless eternity. It is life's instinct and environment, and human society's instinct and environment. To realize it or not realize it makes an enormous difference, even a decisive difference. The Indians realize it, and they can make us know.

The traditional Indian sees the work of the Great Spirit in every expression of life upon the Earth Mother. Such a reverence for the environment convinced the whiteman that the Native American was given to the worship of idols and graven images, a primitive man confused and frightened by a hierarchy of many gods.

The American Indian traditionalist believes that the Great Spirit may express Himself in many ways and may appear in a variety of forms during the vision quest; but, the Amerindian believes in only one Supreme Being. The Native American also believes that the essence of the Great Spirit's power flows through all living things. Regrettably, only a few of the early settlers were able to discern the distinction between witnessing God's work in all of life and worshiping elemental nature forces.

In 1586, Thomas Heriot, an erudite mathematician who became proficient in the tongues of many different tribes, reported: "[The Indians] believe that there is a Supreme God who has existed for all eternity."

David Zeisberger, a Moravian missionary, translated scriptural texts for the Algonquin tribes and was proficient in several native languages. In 1779, from his years of personal contact with several Amerindian nations, he wrote: "They believe and have from time immemorial believed that there is an Almighty Being who has created heaven and earth and man and all things else. This they have learned from their ancestors."

"You didn't try to understand our prayers," Walking Buffalo complained in *Tatana Mani, Walking Buffalo of the Stonies.* "When we sang our praises to the sun or moon or wind, you said we were worshipping idols. Without understanding, you condemned us as lost souls just because our form of worship was different from yours. We saw the Great Spirit's work in almost everything: sun, moon, trees, wind, and mountains. Sometimes we approached him through these things. Was that so bad? I think we have a true belief in the supreme being, a stronger faith than that of most whites who have called us pagans."

The inclination to condemn the American Indian as a lost soul has not been eliminated from the contemporary scene. When I told a prominent southwestern historian the theme of my book, he snorted skeptically and told me that any shreds of religious thought that the Indian might evidence had been adapted from the whiteman.

"The Indian is a notorious borrower," he went on. "At the time of the whiteman's advent to this nation, the Indian was little more than an animal. He was totally incapable of abstract thought. After so many years of the early missionaries pounding stories of Christianity into their heads, the Indians finally caught on, called God the Great Spirit, and tried to say that they had always believed in such a supreme being. The early Indians were interested in physical survival, not spirituality. Every bit of religious philosophy you'll turn up can be traced back to the early Christian missionaries."

Prejudice is a difficult stain to remove from anyone's eyes, but the journals of the earliest whitemen on our continent tell us that the

American Indians believed in a Supreme Being long before the European set his plow in the ground and his church steeples in the air.

Edward Winslow, who accompanied the first colonists to land at Plymouth Rock and who negotiated with Chief Massasoit during the English's initial attempt to explore the interior, reported that the Indians were pleased to learn that the God of the Christians was so very much like their own Kiehtan, creator of all things, who dwelt on high in the western skies.

In a letter dated August 16, 1683, William Penn noted that the Indians in Pennsylvania believed in a Supreme Being and in immortality.

In 1790, Red Jacket, a Seneca chief, made the following remarks to a group of white religionists.

> Brother! You say there is but one way to worship and serve the Great Spirit. If there is but one religion, why do you white people differ so much about it? Why not all agree, as you can all read the [Bible]?
>
> Brother! We do not understand these things. We are told that your religion was given to your forefathers and has been handed down, father to son. We also have a religion which was given to our forefathers, and has been handed down to us, their children. We worship that way. It teaches us to be thankful for all the favors we receive, to love each other, and to be united. We never quarrel about religion.
>
> Brother! The Great Spirit made us all. But he has made a great difference between his white and red children. He has given us a different complexion and different customs. To you he has given the arts: to these he has not opened our eyes. . . . Since he has made so great a difference between us in other things, why may not we conclude that he has given us a different religion, according to our understanding?

"According to our understanding," Red Jacket said, and how many whitemen will concede even today in our era of expanding awareness that the native peoples just might have had a clearer understanding of the teachings of the Great Spirit than did the Western religionists?

The German ethnologist Ivar Lissner maintains that "there once existed a universal, primordial religion, and this primordial religion, far from gaining in strength, has become more and more atrophied." Lissner writes:

> Even in recent years, people of the West believed that mankind had moved upward in its religious beliefs, on an evolutionary spiral which began in earliest times with superstition, mingled with sorcery and magic, to the triumphant evolution of monotheism. This theory held that as man became more civilized he came to see more and more clearly that magic was false and at last reached the highest level of monotheism or belief in one God. Yet. . . a belief in a single supreme deity and creator is found among all the ancient peoples whom we in our arrogance call primitive.

Lissner contends that our continued existence and survival on this planet depend "...on the extent to which the world is guarded and controlled by men of spirituality." We must never cease to reflect upon existence, God, and goodness; we must never permit the arts to die; we must not forsake the heritage of spirituality that has been bequeathed to us over hundreds of thousands of years; we must not allow the materialist, the pure technologist, the rivalry in the exact sciences to dictate the fate of humanity. We must be guided by "great, universal minds which are close to the secrets of the transcendental and throw more into the scales than mere weight of technological progress."

The return of medicine power and the resurrection of the Great Spirit may well be occurring now in an effort to balance the cosmic scales against the dross of materialism. Those transcendental elements which blend together in some spiritually indefinable way to form medicine power may well be the peculiar mystical experience and the proper spiritual path for our continent.

The most essential elements of medicine power are:

The vision quest, with its emphasis on self-denial and spiritual discipline, extended to a lifelong pursuit of wisdom of body and soul.

A reliance upon one's personal visions and dreams to provide one's direction on the path of life.

A search for personal songs to enable one to attune oneself to the primal sound, the cosmic vibration of the Great Spirit.

A belief in a total partnership with the world of spirits and the ability to make personal contact with grandfathers and grandmothers who have changed planes of existence.

The possession of a non-linear time sense.

A receptivity to the evidence that the essence of the Great Spirit may be found in everything.

A reverence and a passion for the Earth Mother, the awareness of one's place in the web of life, and one's responsibility toward all plant and animal life.

A total commitment to one's beliefs that pervades every aspect of one's life and enables one truly to walk in balance.

3
The Vision Quest

When I first asked Dallas Chief Eagle if he had undertaken the vision quest when he was a young man, he quickly replied that he had not. Then, a few moments later, he interrupted our conversation to say: "I have to be perfectly truthful with you, Brad. I forgot what your purpose is in this book you are writing. Yes, I had a vision quest, but I will not comment on it."

I thanked the Sioux chief for his honesty, then asked him: "I realize such things must be kept in secret, but could you tell me if there would still be Indian youths at Rosebud or Pine Ridge who would practice the vision quest today?"

"Yes, definitely," Dallas Chief Eagle answered, "and I wish more youth would, because the vision quest teaches one simplicity, humility, and it certainly adjusts one's attitudes in a spiritual way.

"I think all youths—non-Indian as well as Indian—who have reached puberty should go on a vision quest. Isaac, Abraham, and Jacob went on vision quests. Moses went on a vision quest and obtained the Ten Commandments. Christ himself went on a vision quest for forty days. The term 'vision quest' wasn't used, but we are talking about the same thing."

The vision quest, during which the seeker goes into the wilderness alone to receive a spirit guardian and secret name, constitutes the very essence of medicine power. With its emphasis on individualism and the sacredness of personal visions, the vision quest supplies us with both a prototype of the revelatory experience and a demonstration of the peculiar mystical experience that is most efficacious for our hemisphere.

Don Wanatee, Mesquakie: "This is the time for seeking a definite way whereby you can actually commit yourself to the tribe and to the tribe's beliefs. The tribe depends on you, and you depend on the tribe. When you become older, you must go out and fast for four days and keep on fasting until you get the power. Then it is up to you to distribute this power among your people so they can live a better life, so they can be helped, so they can achieve something and you can be strong.

"I must have been about three or four years old when my great-grandfather introduced me to the Mesquakie tradition [the vision quest]. I remember him sitting there singing. I couldn't sing the songs, because they hadn't really been taught to me yet, but I could tell that they were meaningful to me. I sat there with a gourd, and I remember people dancing, the high shrill of the flute, the cadence of the drum.

"I still maintain [the Mesquakie tradition], because my father followed it, my grandfather followed it, my great-grandfather taught me. That is why I believe very much in the Mesquakie religion and no other, because it was given to us to cherish as a way of life.

"I believe in the [vision quest], that there is a Higher Being to tell you what to do, to tell you this is the way you must help your people, help your family, help your tribe. Yes, I believe in that."

As a young boy, Fay Clark was adopted by Chief Michael Red Cloud of the Winnebagos of Wisconsin. Fay lived among the Winnebagos for two years, and his foster father convinced him to participate in the puberty rite:

> I wouldn't have been quite thirteen. We were given preliminary tutoring for several weeks on what to expect and what was expected of us. Then we were asked to go out into the woods and pick a spot where there was a stream. We were told that we must not bring food or seek out berries or any kind of food. We were also told that we must not seek shelter, but must remain exposed to the elements, to the rain or to the sun. We were to weaken our bodies and to continue praying at least three times a day for our guide.
>
> . . . We prayed to Manitou, the Supreme Being.
>
> The main thought behind the rite is to completely exhaust the body as quickly as possible. One of the exercises the Winnebagos suggested was to find a place where there were rocks, so that we might pick them up and run with them from one place to another. Make a pile one place, then pick them up and carry them back again, repeating the process again and again.

> You see, this exercise enabled one to busy his conscious mind with a monotonous physical activity while the subconscious mind was concentrating on the attainment of one's guide.
>
> After a while, one would begin to see wildlife that would seemingly become friendlier. After a time, some creature would approach, as if to offer itself as a totem, or guide. It could be a bird, a chipmunk, a gopher, a badger. If the boy were very hungry, and if he were afraid of staying out in the wilderness alone, he could accept the first creature that approached and say that he had found his guide. But we were taught that if we could endure, Manitou, or one of his representatives in human form, would appear and talk to us.
>
> I spent twelve days fasting and awaiting my guide. I had many creatures, including a beautiful deer, come up to me and allow me to pet them. The deer, especially, wanted to stay. But I had been told that if I did not want to accept a form of life that offered itself to me, I should thank it for coming, tell it of its beauty, its strength, its intelligence, but tell it also that I was seeking one greater.
>
> On the twelfth day, an illuminated form appeared before me. Although it seemed composed primarily of light, it did have features and was clothed in a long robe.
>
> "You I have waited for," I said. And it replied: "You have sought me, and you I have sought." Then it faded away.
>
> On the evening that each boy was required to appear before the Winnebago council to tell of his experience, my guide was accepted as genuine. And I don't think there is any way that any young boy could have fooled that tribal council. They knew when he had had a real experience and when he had used something as an excuse to get back to the reservation and get something to eat.
>
> One thing that we were taught is that we must never call upon our guides until we had exhausted every bit of physical energy and mental resource possible. Then, after we had employed every last ounce of our own reserve, we might call upon our guide and it would appear.

The personal revelatory experience received during the vision quest becomes the fundamental guiding force in any traditional American Indian's medicine power. The dogma of tribal rituals and the religious expressions of others become secondary to the guidance one receives from one's personal visions.

The vision quest is basic to all native North American religious experience, but one may certainly see similarities between the proud Indian youth presenting himself to the Great Spirit as helpless, shelterless, and humble and the supplicants of Western occultism and Christianity, fasting, flagellating, and prostrating themselves in monastic cells. In Christianity, of course, the questing mystic kneels before a personal deity and beseeches insight from the Son of God, whom he hopes to please with his example of piety and self-sacrifice. In Native American medicine, as in occultism, the power, the mana, granted by the vision quest comes from a vast and impersonal repository of spiritual energy, and each recipient of medicine power becomes his own priest, his own shaman, who will be guided by guardian spirits and by insights into the workings of the cosmos granted to him by visions sent from the Great Spirit.

The vision quest is the Native American's first communion. Far from being a goal achieved, the vision quest marks the beginning of the traditional Indian's lifelong search for knowledge and wisdom. Nor are the spiritual mechanics of the vision quest ignored once the youth has established contact with the guardian spirit and with the power which are to aid him in the shaping of his destiny. At any stress period of his life, the traditional American Indian may go into the wilderness to fast and to seek insight into the particular problems that beset him.

As Hartley Burr Alexander writes in *The World's Rim*:

> The seeker goes forth solitary, if a man, carrying his pipe and with an offering of tobacco, and there in the wilderness, alone, he chants his song and utters his prayer while he waits, fasting, such revelation as the Powers may grant. Perhaps as evidence of the intensity of his need he sacrifices a dear possession or offers the blood of his own body that the Ministers of the Great Spirit may the more readily respond. The Indian prophets, men such as Tecumseh, Keokuk, Smohalla, Wovoka, have almost invariably secured their revelations in this manner; and Indian tradition is filled with tales of men and women who have undertaken the sojourn in solitude, their days in the wilderness, not alone for their individual need but for the welfare of the whole people.

Dallas Chief Eagle has already pointed out that the inspired prophets of the Jewish and Christian traditions have undertaken the wilderness sojourn in the same kind of seeking of the Great Spirit's revelations. The difference in the traditions lies in the fact that whereas the Christian or Jew accepts the idea that *the chosen* of God have gone into the wilderness to seek illumination, the American Indian has made the vision quest a part of the life of *everyone* who seeks medicine power. Members of nearly every Christian congregation will assume that their clerical shepherd received some kind of "call" that led to the ministry, but the vast majority of the congregation were born into their faith and would undoubtedly be puzzled by anyone asking them if they had received a "call" to become a member of that church body. The American Indian does not wait for some cosmic signal to be summoned into communion with a higher intelligence. The Native American goes into the wilderness to await and to confront the vision and the guardian spirit.

The matter of the guardian spirit will seem but a fairy tale to the skeptic, while to the orthodox religionist, who may cherish a belief in angels, this American Indian belief will smack of pagan mysticism. The psychologist may tell us that men and women in isolation will often hallucinate supernatural helpers. However, the concept of ultra-physical beings materializing to assist us in times of crisis appears to be universal.

Messenger entities, with a more than casual interest in us, may come from the Great Spirit to perform precisely the functions which they claim. They may be externalized projections of our own High Self (our superego) which appear to help us help ourselves. They are a manifestation in which the Great Spirit reveals itself to us in an appropriate form that will permit us to perceive the revelation in the most meaningful manner.

Fay Clark told me that his guardian spirit has responded to his calls for help and that on two occasions it has appeared to warn him of approaching danger. Whether the ostensible spirit was an independent intelligent entity concerned about Fay's welfare or whether the manifestation was due to Fay's superconscious level of mind receiving information through other than sensory means and externalizing the knowledge as a warning spirit, he did not hesitate to act upon the information received.

Dr. Walter Houston Clark told me: "I have learned things about myself and the mystical consciousness from visionary experience under the influence of psychedelic chemicals, as at an Indian peyote ceremony, for example. But any figures I have seen in such states, I have always assumed to have been symbols created by my unconscious, rather than coming from an intelligence in another plane of being. Nevertheless, those who have received messages from cowled figures, angels, or venerable men in dreams and visions and then find that these messages contain verifiable truths should treat these figures with respect, whatever their origin."

The traditional American Indian certainly treats his guardian spirit with respect, and he uses the information given to him in dreams and in visions as lessons about himself to be used in the most effective performance of his personal medicine. If one feels more comfortable considering the guardian to be an externalized image of the High Self, which the percipient receives as a by-product of the illumination of the vision quest, it would probably not greatly affect one's medicine power.

To emphasize the uniqueness of the vision quest as the fundamental guiding force in Native American medicine is to underscore certain universal aspects of the experience and to invite comparisons with the *samadhi* of the Yogi, the *satori* of the Zen Buddhist, Dr. Raymond Bucke's Cosmic Consciousness, and the ecstasy of the Christian mystic. In the chapter "Basic Mystical Experience" in his *Watcher on the Hills*, Dr. Raynor C. Johnson named the following seven characteristics of illumination, which are listed here with comments directed toward our analysis of the vision quest of the American Indian:

The Appearance of Light. One instantly thinks of Paul (né Saul) on the road to Damascus being struck blind by the sudden appearance of a bright light; but, the guardian spirit also manifests as a light being.

Ecstasy, Love, Bliss. The traditional Native American, stereotypically regarded as stoical and unfeeling, regarded the vision quest as a supreme emotional experience.

The Approach to Oneness. The very essence of the traditional way of life is the awareness that one is a part of the universe and the universe is a part of oneself.

Insights Given. The seeker receives valuable insights, a guardian, and a secret name.

Effect on Health and Vitality. After the illumination experience, the percipient—after fasting for several days and depleting all physical strength through monotonous tasks designed to quiet the conscious mind—would feel invigorated and would walk back to the council in full stride to recount the vision.

Sense of Time Obscured. Because the Native American is not enslaved by linear time, this seems less dramatic to the traditional American Indian than to other recipients of illumination.

Effects on Living. The receiving of the personal vision serves as the traditional Indian's support throughout life and is incorporated into a world-view with total commitment.

"To receive visions [beyond the vision quest experience] is a great thing," Iron Eyes Cody said. "But it is not always easy to have visions. I was in the sweat lodge a couple of years ago. My son was heating the rocks. A man passed out. My son was darn near passing out. Another man was coughing so that he couldn't sing with the rest of us. Then he saw his grandmother [that is, his grandmother's spirit form] in a dark place in the sweat lodge. Now, you have to believe this, because a vision is a matter of power of the mind. Visions come. You can see them. But you have to be strong-minded.

"My wife didn't tell you this, but a couple of years ago we had a Yuwipi meeting right here in the darkroom of my photography studio. We were talking about healing a woman. There were different ones here. Eagle Feather, the medicine man, came here to conduct the Yuwipi meeting. My wife was sitting next to the woman to be healed. The drummer was going; we were chanting.

"When we stopped, something hit my wife in the lap. When we turned on the lights, we saw that it was a bundle of feathers that had been on the other side of the room. Nobody could have got there to grab those feathers. Eagle Feather was by the altar in the middle. My son, Rocky Boy, and I were singing and drumming. Nobody could have got by us. The power of our Yuwipi happening made that bunch of feathers come and land in my wife's lap. After everyone saw what had happened, a lot of people told what they had felt and saw while we were in darkness. Magic is a strong power."

How does one best acquire the visions that lead to strong medicine power? There is the vision quest, of course, but are there other techniques which might encourage the advent of meaningful visions?

Don Wilkerson: "There are certain ceremonies—and you can buy records of them—such as the Navajo *Yeibichai,* that are very hypnotic. If you listen to them, you will discover what they can do to you. Listening to a Yeibichai in a darkened, quiet room is a very, very moving experience. The tone is very high-pitched and chillingly done. It'll do it to you!"

Iron Eyes Cody: "If the songs are sung properly, they can work great magic. I had been a technical advisor in films for years when Cecil B. De Mille, during the filming of *The Unconquered,* said to me, 'You speak the Seneca language. You know the Seneca songs. I want you to play Red Corn, as well as be technical advisor.'

"But these things must be done correctly. In *A Man Called Horse,* I was told to jump up and down and throw powder in Richard Harris's face before the Sun Dance. I said no. I am a Yuwipi man of the medicine society of the Yuwipi. It is not done that way. An old medicine man 'way up in his nineties, Richard Fools Crow, said, 'I'm glad you said that, Iron Eyes. You stick to it.'

"I told the director that I would rather just quit than be unfaithful to my Yuwipi society. So he said, 'All right, let's see you do it your way.'

"So I did it the very calm way and went through the ceremony, putting the eagle claws and the skewers through the whiteman's chest muscles, singing a song that defied the whiteman's magic. But the whiteman's power showed that he could do the Sun Dance, too. So at the end of the dance, I show that I admire the whiteman. I come in singing a blessing song.

"I would never have sung proper ceremonial songs in some of the terrible pictures I have been in. I have been made to play hateful killers, and I would not further debase my people by permitting true ceremonial songs to be sung in these movies.

"Walt Disney put me under contract for four years when he was filming the Daniel Boone television series. [This early series starred Dewey Martin and should not be confused with the later series starring Fess Parker.] Walt told me that he wanted me to teach some of those Indians in North Carolina to sing an old ceremonial song. But the song I taught to them was just a common work song. I couldn't give the true ceremonial song for this series.

". . . I did a picture called *The Great Sioux Massacre.* I played Crazy Horse, a great man who sang strange songs, a man who saw visions. Things came to Crazy Horse that no one could explain. I read the book about him by Mari Sandoz. I talked to people up there in Rosebud, Pine Ridge, South Dakota. Nobody knew about the man, but they knew his ways and they followed them. He was a great man, and we use him now in songs. In this picture they wanted me to be Crazy Horse singing the old Sun Dance songs. I wouldn't do it.

"But when *A Man Called Horse* came along, I did sing the sun vow song. At first, as I said, I would not. I did not want to ridicule my people. But when the director let me play the part in a spiritual way—the way I wanted to play it—that song came out of me as soon as I walked into the lodge. I did this great song—the *Wakan Tanka*—with feeling. I didn't see a camera. I heard nothing that was going on around me. I just went through the whole ceremonial song. The *Wakan Tanka* is not a song we sing every day. It is sung only at the Sun Dance, and this was the picture in which it was to come out for all to hear."

Black Elk, great medicine man of the Oglala Sioux, told how he began to sing his vision song when he felt that spirits from the outer world wished to speak to him. After chanting the words of his sacred song

["Behold! A sacred voice is calling you! All over the sky a sacred voice is calling!"] an uncounted number of repetitions, the two men of his great vision appeared to him with a relevant message.

In his monumental work, *Battle for the Mind,* and again in a lecture entitled "The Physiology of Faith," Dr. William Sargant discusses the two main ways in which revelatory insight may be acquired by the mystic.

The first method involves overexciting the nervous system "by means of drumming, dancing and music of various kinds, by the rhythmic repetition of stimuli and by the imposing of emotionally charged mental conflicts needing urgent resolution," and would seem to be referring to the revelations acquired by involvement in singing or dancing the Yeibichai, the Wakan Tanka, or any other particularly dramatic ceremony.

The other method inhibits most of the ordinary voluntary and even involuntary thoughts and activities of the higher nervous system: "One tries to put oneself artificially in what is now increasingly called a state of 'sensory deprivation.' "

Dr. Sargant seems to be referring to such spiritual techniques as those employed in the vision quest when he goes on to state:

> In states of contemplation and mysticism. . . the individual has deliberately to learn. . . how to empty his mind of all extraneous matters, and generally to center his thoughts, if he is finally thinking actively at all, on some subject on which he desires to obtain new enlightenment. . . . What then seems to happen is that, as the brain becomes more and more severely inhibited as regards its normal functions, one gets a greater and greater concentration on the one thing that matters at the time, or, as Henry Maudsley put it, 'extreme activity of one part of the brain and extreme lassitude of the rest'. . . . Suddenly the particular god. . . being concentrated on is felt actually to enter the person and become a very part of himself. . . . Impressions made on the brain at such a stage may remain lifelong in their effects, and from that time on, the individual has not the slightest doubt that the possessions or other sensations he experienced. . . were true in fact, despite all other life experiences. . . .

Whether or not one accepts such psychological explanations for revelatory experiences, I believe that one basic question must be answered: Do rituals, drumming, dancing, chanting, fasting, or sensory deprivation induce the vision, or do these devices help enable the vision to occur?

Dr. Robert E.L. Masters and Dr. Jean Houston of the Foundation for Mind Research in New York City have concluded on the basis of hundreds of experiments with normal, healthy persons in the non-drug induction of religious-type experiences in the laboratory that "the brain-mind system has a built-in contact point with what is experienced as God, fundamental reality, or the profoundly sacred." Dr. Houston went on to comment: "The capacity for religious experience—including a deep feeling of unity with the universe—is built into human nature. It's simply a question of opening oneself up."

For many years Twylah Nitsch taught a course in "Seneca Wisdom" at the Human Dimensions Institute in Buffalo, New York. The course dealt with "self-realization, self-control and how to live in harmony with Nature."

According to Twylah:

> The Indians did give instructions that helped one function within his highest intellectual self, which is the spiritual self. If all people would let themselves be guided by their spiritual selves, their material world would be more satisfying.
>
> There is one technique, that of the use of the senses and going into the silence.
>
> If you have a problem, go into the silence—which to me is not meditation. Meditation is only the door to silence, wherein you communicate with the inner self, the spiritual energy that is universal. When you have shut out the external world and are deep in the silence, you work, for instance, with sight. If you do not have success in seeing an image, try the sense of smell.
>
> Some you will hit on something that will be very meaningful, but you must *feel*. You cannot taste unless you feel; you cannot see unless you feel. When you are feeling and raising your emotional level, you tap into the creative self, the highest intellectual self, that which is of God and which is, to the Indian, the universal energy responsible for life.
>
> Whenever I see or hear a prayer written by an Indian that says, "Great Spirit, grant me this or that"—a prayer of supplication—I know that it has been infiltrated with other philosophies. A traditional Indian never asks, never offers prayers of supplication—he only offers prayers of thanks. This is a true, hard fact, and one that is very important to an understanding of medicine.
>
> My grandfather was Moses Shongo, last of the medicine doctors of the Seneca nation. He said that the people of today have not evolved sufficiently enough and intellectually enough to understand the principles of the original people of this country. He said at the end of the Fourth World—which is the world we are in now—there will be a great awakening and we may be able to talk about some of these things. That is why I am beginning to talk a little bit. I think the time is beginning to open up. . . .

> It was not only the young men who sought visions. There was an equality between the sexes. The woman would have to do what she would have to do to live with herself. She could go out and do the same things her own way. This was a personal thing. No one was ever forced to do it. When you felt you were ready, you did it. It was a communion within yourself and with Nature.

"If I am going to seek a vision of enlightenment or direction, then I usually go off by myself and find a place that is comfortable," Sun Bear said. "Sometimes I will take off all my clothing and offer myself to the Great Spirit just as I came into the world. This is the thing that I do when I seek my visions, my medicine counsel."

Black Elk has said, "A man who has a vision is not able to use the power of it until after he has performed the vision on earth for the people to see." He, of course, is not talking about the highly personal insight received during the vision quest, but the great vision that will enable one to become a medicine practitioner and have the strength to cure others and to counsel those in need.

"Of course it was not I who cured," Black Elk qualifies in *Black Elk Speaks.* "It was the power from the outer world, and the visions and ceremonies had only made me like a hole through which the power could come to the two-leggeds. If I thought that I was doing it myself, the hole would close up and no power could come through."

Black Elk's qualifying remarks sound so much like the disclaimers which I have heard from sincere psychic sensitives, mediums, and healers who refuse any personal credit for their feats, but rather refer to themselves as "channels" through which the power may flow. It appears that it may be a universal law of metaphysics that those who are chosen to serve as "holes," as "channels," be ever conscious of the proper perspective in which they are to regard the stewardship of their unique abilities.

"The very fact that you can use medicine power to accomplish something is enough," Sun Bear explained. "You don't have to boast of it or pat yourself on the back. I know one brother who is a medicine person of this area [Nevada] who would boast of his medicine power. He lost his power for a period of time because of this."

Again, like so many accomplished adepts of metaphysics, the sincere practitioner of medicine believes that, from time to time, the essential self, the soul, leaves the physical shell of the body and soars free of time and space to travel other dimensions of existence and to receive spiritual insights not possible even in deep meditation or in going into the silence.

Black Elk, for example, was a boy of nine when he heard voices telling him "it was time" just before he received his great vision. He fell ill, was taken out of his body by two men who told him they were to take him to his grandfathers. In the land of the spirits, Black Elk received the great vision that was to sustain him all of his life. When he was returned to his body, his parents greeted the first flutter of his eyelids with great joy. He had been lying as if dead for twelve days.

When he was with a wild west show in Paris, the homesick Black Elk was partaking of a meal in the home of a family who had befriended him, when, as he sat at the table, he looked up at the ceiling and it seemed to be moving. Then he was soaring through the clouds, traveling over the big water of the Atlantic, crossing over New York City, the Missouri River, the Black Hills, until he hovered over his home at Pine Ridge. While he viewed the camps below him from his remarkable vantage point, he was able to see things which he was able to verify when he returned to the land of the Lakotas several days later. Again, he had lain as dead—this time for three days in the home of the solicitous French family.

In 1890, two years before the tragic massacre at Wounded Knee, Black Elk had an out-of-body experience while dancing, and he returned from the land of the spirits with the design for the holy shirts, the shirts to be used while participating in the Ghost Dance.

The Ghost Dance was originally the vision of Wovoka, a Paiute medicine man who was adept at sleight-of-hand magic, impressed with the Christian stories of Jesus' Second Coming, and sorrowed by the state of poverty and despair to which the Indian nations had been reduced. Wovoka received a messianic charge while in a fever-induced trance and awakened with a long-sought prophecy of redemption for the Indian, a promise of the termination of white domination, and a hope for the regeneration of the despoiled earth and the return of the buffalo. Wovoka had no further use for the magic tricks he had used to supplement his medicine. He was imbued with power, and he would work for peace between the Indian and non-Indian.

Wovoka advocated a code of conduct established upon the principles of peace, brotherhood, forbearance, and nonviolence. Handsome Lake, Smohalla, and John Slocum (founder of Shakerism) had preached similar principles, but they had been prophets. Wovoka told his followers that he was Jesus once again upon the earth. Tragically, the hypnotic manifestation of the *dance-in-a-circle,* which Wovoka brought back from Spirit to permit every participant to mingle with the ghosts of loved ones, evolved into the

Sioux Nation's Ghost Dance, the *wana ghi wa chipi,* which spun the Indians away from their aspirations of a bloodless victory and lead them in confusion to the bloody massacre at Wounded Knee.

In some cases, dancers wearing Ghost Shirts, said to be able to turn the whiteman's bullets to water, forgot that the dance was one of peace and left the circle to take full advantage of their supposed invulnerability. In other cases, fearful and suspicious whites simply could not believe that Indians could dance for peace as well as for war. This unfortunate state of tension resulted in the terrible murders at Wounded Knee. Wovoka became ill when he learned of the slaughter. He had died and gone to heaven to bring back a dance of peace, a dance which told the living that the dead would not forsake them, a dance that would make the land green and free once again. God had told him to tell his children not to fight, not to kill.

"Wovoka was a healer, a man of great magic," Iron Eyes Cody said. "We know that maybe at the beginning he fooled some of the people with tricks, but we have to say that Wovoka was a spiritual man.

"When I was a boy, I was with Tim McCoy. Tim went out to appear in Nevada and to meet a heavyset old preacher. They had a picture taken together. The old preacher—that was Wovoka—told me that he had believed what the Great Spirit had told him. He said that he didn't go into eating hallucinogenic herbs or anything like that. He had done everything through his medicine power."

I asked Iron Eyes if Wovoka still identified himself with Jesus at that time.

"Yes, he did," Iron Eyes answered. "It is too bad, but Wovoka's descendants don't even come to our powwows. It's like they don't even want to admit that they are Indians, you know."

Andrew Vidovitch, Wovoka's son-in-law, passed on in the spring of 1972, leaving, it appears, no spiritual heir to the vision that Wovoka had for his people [Wovoka died in 1932]. Vidovitch's active participation in the filming of *Billy Jack* and his willingness to commit an accurate representation of the Ghost Dance to film may indicate that his medicine told him that cinematic imagery might be an ideal method of preserving his father-in-law's vision for millions of today's youth and for those yet unborn.

I was fortunate in being able to talk with Mamie Babcock, a sister-in-law of Andrew Vidovitch.

Mamie Babcock: "Andy told everyone about it. He was so wrapped up in it. Every time we came down for a holiday, why, the main subject was this thing that you are talking about now."

About the Great Spirit and the Ghost Dance vision?

Mrs. Babcock: "Yes, he always mentioned the Great Spirit. And he actually lived his belief, you know what I mean?"

He lived a completely spiritual life?

Mrs. Babcock: "Yes. He was always a good, clean-cut, spiritual man. I am so sorry that you couldn't have got here before he died. It was a wonderful thing to hear him tell about it all."

Is there anyone else in the family who will carry on Wovoka's vision?

Mrs. Babcock: "No. Among the members of the family there doesn't seem to be any interest in the old traditions. Most of them couldn't go back that far. They attend Christian churches. I go to church. It is hard getting our young people to go to church. It is like telling them to take castor oil or something.

"But, oh, Andy used to speak of Wovoka all the time. Many an evening when we came down here, he told us about it. My grandchildren will always remember Grandpa Andy talking about Wovoka. Wovoka and the Great Spirit."

Although it seems rather sad that Wovoka no longer has a spiritual heir in his own bloodline, his vision is being danced time after time at innumerable Native American gatherings. The Ghost Dance mythos, with its melding of Christianity and the old traditions, is one of the progenitors of the contemporary Native American Church.

4

Healing with Prayers, Herbs, and Crystals

> Dallas, Texas—the National Institute of Mental Health, a United States federal agency that funds numerous projects to improve the delivery of psychiatric services, is paying six Navajo medicine men on an Arizona reservation to teach twelve young Indians the elaborate ceremonies that often cure the mental ailments of Navajos.
>
> And, according to a conventionally-trained psychiatrist involved in the program, there is every indication that the trainees will become effective psycho-therapists, able to meet the mental health needs of a growing Navajo population that finds Anglo psychiatry ineffective.
>
> The psychiatrist, Dr. Robert L. Bergman of the Indian Health Service in Window Rock, Arizona, described the unusual program May 4 at the annual meeting of the American Psychiatric Association here.
>
> The program is an example of a growing awareness among Western-trained psychiatrists that the treatment for many mental illnesses must meet the cultural expectations of the patient and that virtually every culture has given rise to healers of some sort who are as effective in dealing with mental problems among their people as psychiatrists among Westerners.
>
> Dr. Bergman said the Navajo program began when Indian reservation leaders decided something had to be done to increase the supply of medicine men. The remaining medicine men were becoming quite old, and few young men were able to assume the economic hardship of several years in training, traditionally in apprenticeship to be established medicine men. . . . [*New York Times*, May 6, 1972]

The unique school for medicine men is located at Rough Rock, Arizona, a community near the center of the Navajo Reservation, approximately seventy miles from its nearest border. It is a part of the Rough Rock Demonstration School, the first community-controlled Indian school. Since the very idea of a school for medicine men seems so representative of some of the things that are occurring to herald the rebirth of medicine power and the resurrection of the Great Spirit, I considered myself extremely fortunate when Dr. Robert L. Bergman, Chief of the Mental Health Service, (the psychiatrist who has been working with medicine people in Rough Rock) granted me an interview:

Dr. Bergman, I am certain that a lot of serious-minded people must ask you this question: How can you be working to promote mental health when you are involved in a project that appears to be a retreat to superstition, a step backward culturally?

Dr. Robert L. Bergman: "I usually answer that question by pointing out that the proper definition of the word superstition is, *my* knowledge, *your* belief, *his* superstition. Superstition is a word which conveys a lot of things without conveying a whole lot of information."

You are saying, then, that superstition is a pejorative term used to express disapproval of someone else's system of beliefs.

Dr. Bergman: "You could equally well refer—as I suppose some people do—to the superstitious belief of millions of Americans in the presence on Earth at one partcular time of a person who was both human and God."

How did the older traditionalists feel about the idea of cutting through the many years of apprenticeship and turning out medicine men in a school, à la the Western tradition of mass education?

Dr. Bergman: "Well, the school doesn't really offer any short-cuts. It is taking students a little bit longer than we had expected, probably because they are spending nearly full time on their studies, but it still takes a long time. And the ones who have graduated have only learned two ceremonies each. There is a lot of grousing right now by those graduates, who are complaining that they wanted to learn more and that they wish they had been permitted to stay in school longer. At any rate, it took them three and four years to learn just those two ceremonies, so you cannot say the school is mass production. And I should point out that the only part that is done in school proper is my work with them. The ceremonies are learned in a traditional way through apprenticeship in the homes of medicine men and in the places where they perform ceremonies.

"I don't know how many ceremonies there are, but the important ones last five or nine nights, and they are difficult and elaborate to a degree approached among us conventional doctors only by open heart surgery.

"A major sing, to be properly performed, demands the presence of the entire extended family, and many other of the patient's social connections. The patient's immediate family must feed all of these people for days. Many of the people present are employed in important roles in the ceremony, such as chanting, public speaking, dancing in costume, leading group discussions, and other activities which are more or less ritualized. For the singer-medicine man, the performance requires the letter-perfect performance of up to one hundred hours of ritual chant—a feat which might be compared to a perfect recitation of the New Testament from memory. In addition, the medicine man must produce a number of beautiful and ornate sand paintings, recite the myth connected with the ceremony, and manage a very large and difficult group process."

I appreciate that clarification, Doctor. Can you tell me what would be the average age of the student and the average age of the graduate at Rough Rock's medicine school?

Dr. Bergman: "I've never figured that out. Let's see, the students who just graduated, I imagine, would average about fifty years old. The faculty currently averages about eighty-five. These studies are not usually undertaken early in life, although there are exceptions."

Would it be fair to say that as with the holy men of other traditions—I am thinking, for example, of the Zen Buddhist priest—that these studies might be best undertaken when some of the other affairs of life, such as rearing a family, earning a livelihood, have more or less been put to one side?

Dr. Bergman: "Yes, that is quite correct in general. I think in older times the studies for the position of medicine man were really taken up in adolescence or in middle age. We had one adolescent student, but he couldn't stand the strain. Now we have another adolescent in our new bunch, and there are many men who are in their thirties. I think the average age of the present group of students is around forty."

I have found, after interviewing medicine people from many different tribes, that one criterion for the role of shaman, or medicine man, is that somewhere in childhood or adolescence, the individual undergoes a seizure, an intense fever wherein he appears to die, or a high fever that brings about convulsions. Would this criterion hold for any of the medicine students at Rough Rock now?

Dr. Bergman: "No, you are talking about shamans, and these guys are not seers. Navajo practitioners generally fall into three categories. There are the herbalists, who know a variety of medicinal plants to be used primarily for symptomatic relief. Then they have the diagnosticians, who are shamans who work by inspiration and employ such techniques as hand trembling, crystal gazing, or star gazing. These diagnosticians divine the nature and the cause of an illness and make the proper referral to a member of the third and highest status group, the singers. These men—and I will use the terms "ceremonialist," "medicine man," and "singer" synonymously—do the true curative work. The school at Rough Rock seeks to train singers, medicine men."

So the medicine people here are medicine *in a sense approaching our Western meaning, in that they are being trained primarily to help with healing physical and mental ills, rather than developing seership.*

Dr. Bergman: "Yes, these fellows are learning to cure; they are not learning to divine."

[Traditionally, "medicine power" provides insights, strength, and spiritual power, but this medicine may not include the ability to heal. However, one who has developed a high degree of medicine power generally discovers that the ability to heal is a natural byproduct of total spiritual attunement. Some Native Americans favor the term "sacred doctor" to describe such an individual and to distinguish him from a "medicine man," who may have the ability to heal but who has not developed his full spiritual potential. Ivar Lissner defines a shaman as one "who knows how to deal with spirits and influence them. . . . The essential characteristic of the shaman is his excitement, his ecstasy and trancelike condition. . . . (The elements which constitute this ecstasy are) a form of self-severance from mundane existence, a state of heightened sensibility and spiritual awareness. The shaman loses outward consciousness and becomes inspired or enraptured. While in this state of enthusiasm he sees dreamlike apparitions, hears voices, and receives visions of truth. More than that, his soul sometimes leaves his body to go wandering."]

You have mentioned that these students spend quite a bit of time interpreting their dreams.

Dr. Bergman: "Yes, this is in relation to the curative aspects of their dreams. Again, they are not using their dreams to predict the future of the tribe or their patients. They regard their dreams as do I—as an indication of their own state of well-being. Or a patient's dreams are an important indication of how he is doing."

This correlates with psychoanalytic procedure. Many therapists have mentioned how their dreams may give them insights into a patient's progress, and, in some cases, how their dreams may seem to intertwine with those of a patient.

Dr. Bergman: "Yes. I meet with the students one full day every two weeks, and we spend a great deal of time on dreams. I admit that Navajo metapsychology still largely eludes me, but I have learned that they know about the dynamic interpretation of dreams. We have been pleased to discover that all of us follow the same custom in regard to our dreams. We all spend our first waking moments in the morning contemplating and interpreting our dreams."

Although you have said that you have not used any of the Navajo ceremonies yourself, would you say that you have become more sympathetic toward there being a presence, an atmosphere, another order, a separate reality at work in these ceremonies?

Dr. Bergman: "Yes, I can conceive of that. I am not sure it is necessary to explain what happens, though. I am more impressed with the need of supernatural explanations for some of the things that the shaman can do; but, again, it is just one of those things where I don't think it matters a whole lot. It seems to me to be the kind of question that seems fascinating, but when you really get into it, it isn't. At least it doesn't fascinate me to try to bring together scientific principles for everything that happens in life. I think that there are some things that are better looked at from an artistic, aesthetic, religious point of view. An attempt to try to bring them into one system with a scientific analysis of natural phenomena is kind of hopeless and kind of boring.

"Non-Navajo explanations of why their rituals help anyone tend to be rather offensive to the medicine men themselves. The Navajo medicine men just do not make so much of the distinctions among different levels of reality as the non-Indian. They reject as stupid and destructive any attempt to translate their words into ordinary language. Though it may seem to me that their myths and chants are symbols of human social and psychological forces and events, they would consider such statements as silly and as totally missing the point.

"A one-hundred-year-old medicine man named Thomas Largewhiskers said to me: 'I don't know what you learned from books, but the most important thing I learned from my grandfathers was that there is a part of the mind that we don't really know about and that it is that part that is most important in whether we become sick or remain well.' "

It seems to me that you have come to accept the value of both Indian and non-Indian medicine, and like a good Yankee pragmatist, you utilize both of them. Would that be a fair statement?

Dr. Bergman: "Well, this is necessary in psychiatry. In psychiatry we use a kind of mythology of the mind. From the rigorous scientific point of view, the mind is probably a rather flimsy construct at best. We have a very elaborate dynamic model of the mind that we use constantly, but which doesn't coincide with any neuroanatomical or physiological stuff that we know. If one can stand to live with those two worlds, he can always add a few more."

What are your plans for the future of the school for medicine men? Will you need to establish any incentive programs to keep the project running?

Dr. Bergman: "No, we don't need any incentive program, but we are going to need funds. There are already several other communities here on the Navajo reservation that are talking about setting up a similar program, and I have had letters from a number of other tribes asking me for my help in setting up a program in their areas. Indian people are getting themselves together, and sooner or later—I hope sooner—probably other communities will want to make application to the National Institute of Mental Health; and if I can, I will help them. I am not part of the NIMH, but being a psychiatrist and working for another branch of the Public Health Service, I can help them prepare applications to get source money."

Have you ever received criticism from orthodox religious groups or from professional medical societies?

Dr. Bergman: "There is a physician who practices in Gallup, New Mexico—which is where I live—who is the son of a Baptist missionary, who wrote to his congressman, saying that we were supporting paganism. The congressman gave us a chance to reply, then used our reply to give the doctor a very firm answer. A faculty member from some small Catholic college wrote to another congressman, complaining that it wasn't right at all for Catholic elementary schoolchildren to be denied federal educational aid, when Navajo priests were being trained by federal money. After three or four days of thought, I managed to come up with a reply that federal aid does go to Catholic medical schools.

"As far as criticism from my colleagues, at the American Psychiatric Association I was called a paternalistic racist."

You have said that your contact with the Navajo singers has caused you to try to act like a medicine man.

Dr. Bergman: "That has to do with my acquiring some of their style of communicating with patients, not in my performing any of their ceremonies. I think I picked up some of their habits of nonverbal communication and some of their attitudes toward patients. The medicine men are extremely modest. They always deny knowing anything, and they almost never make any claims for ever having any successes or having any special knowledge. At the same time, they give a lot of nonverbal clues that they expect a lot of respect. The important thing is that we have made more personal contact with one another. We have shared some of those illuminating experiences when we see what someone really meant by saying or doing something.

"Actually, the major accomplishment of the school for medicine men is that we have really turned out some medicine men. And that was the idea of our project: to replenish the supply of medicine men."

> O you people, be you healed;
> Life anew I bring unto you.
> O you people, be you healed;
> Life anew I bring unto you.
> Through the Great Spirit over all do I this;
> Life anew unto you!
>
> —Lakota holy song

Although the Menninger Foundation of Topeka, Kansas, has announced no plans to convert any of its facilities to a school for medicine men, Douglas Boyd, a research assistant there, was assigned to follow the Shoshone medicine man Rolling Thunder for a year to see what he could learn about Native American approaches to healing.

"Rolling Thunder works on a very powerful kind of archetypal level," said Dr. Irving Oyle, director of a health service in Bolinas, California. "Western medicine can well afford to keep an eye on Rolling Thunder."

"We medicine people see things that others can't see," Rolling Thunder has said. "It's not us that does it, it is the Great Spirit."

Rolling Thunder told a group of assembled psychiatrists, psychologists, and other professional people at the Menninger Foundation that every medicine man has his own medicine. He would not define his approach for them because, "if a medicine man tells what his medicine is, he loses his power."

It has been clear to those who have listened to Rolling Thunder that his work with the ill cannot be separated in his mind from his work as a close observer of the Earth Mother. Medicine people believe that the Great Spirit would never put a disease on this plane of existence without placing the remedy here, too. For centuries, medicine people have made sincere efforts to become brothers with all living things so that they might discern the hidden spirits of the plant world and be able to make remedies which would aid their people.

The twilight-blooming Moon Flower (Jimsonweed) was used as a soothing drug. Once the leaves had been dried, patients would smoke them to treat such ailments as asthma, cholera, and epilepsy. Today the chemicals in this flower are distilled for use in tranquilizers and eye dilations.

Medicine people found that small amounts of mistletoe were effective in treating epilepsy, and the leaves and berries, cooked with rice, formed a poultice used to draw pus from infections.

The Shoshone, Navajo, and Blackfeet chewed stone seed, a common weed of the area, for an oral contraceptive. Modern laboratory analysis has discovered that the plant contains estrogen, the same substance that is used in today's Pill.

Diarrhea was treated by the root of a cherry tree, the leaf of the horsetail weed, and the root of the blackberry.

Indians found an instant Band-Aid in the thick juice of the milkweed plant.

Toothache was dealt with by chewing the root of wild licorice and holding it in the mouth.

Salicylic acid, the basic ingredient of aspirin, can be found in willow bark, the basis of a brew prescribed by medicine people for headaches and for fevers.

Patients with stomach upsets were given swamp root, manzanilla buds, or branches of the juniper.

Soapweed may be used as a shampoo that gives luster to the hair.

An application of the boiled leaves of horse mint makes an excellent acne treatment.

The list of Native American herbal remedies is an extensive one. We may marvel at the ancient medicine people's ability to discern the curative power of roots, leaves, and barks that our modern, sanitary laboratories have since stamped with their seals of approval, but, an herb is, after all, an organic chemical compound and its brew is a recognizable medicine, whether it is steeped over a campfire or bottled in a pharmaceutical plant. The wonder and magic have been removed from something as familiar as a tonic, a syrup, or a chewable bromide. However, we are still curious and fascinated by acts of healing that are undoubtedly even older than the prescribing of herbs and elixirs. We want to know how faith healing, chanting, and the laying on of hands can cure.

Psychiatrist-anthropologist Dr. E. Fuller Torrey has classified what he considers to be the four common components of curing that are utilized by physician-healers all over the world.

The naming process. Since there is nothing more frightening to a patient than the unknown, the very act of giving the illness or complaint a name that fits in with the patient's world view "may activate a series of associated ideas in the patient's mind, producing confession, emotional reaction, and general catharsis."

The personality characteristics of the healer. The doctor-healers who possess the personal qualities of accurate empathy, non-possessive warmth, and genuineness "consistently and convincingly get better results than those who do not possess them."

The patient's expectations. Doctor-healers all over the world use basically the same methods of raising their patients' expectations. The physical stimulus of amulet, rattle, stethoscope, or diploma are common ways in which expectations are increased. It is also a common observation that the farther a patient has to travel to visit the healer, the greater are the chances of a cure.

The doctor-healer's training. Although few cultures other than the Western ones have a regular examination at the end of the training period, all genuine and sincere healers in all cultures undergo rigorous training programs that may last several years.

Dr. Torrey observes that the same techniques of therapy are used by healers regardless of whether one finds them in hogans or in Park Avenue suites. "It is this aspect of therapy that is the most difficult to see in cross-cultural perspective," he comments, "because we would like to believe that the techniques used by Western therapists are 'scientific' and those used by therapists elsewhere are 'magical.'

"In fact, this is wrong. We have failed to see this because we have confused our technology with our techniques; whatever goes on in a modern office must be science, whereas what goes on in a grass hut must be magic. We have also confused education with techniques; we assume that a Ph.D. or M.D. only does scientific things, whereas a person who is illiterate must do magical things. . . . But there is no technique used by Western therapists that is not also found in other cultures."

Dr. Bernard Grad, an associate professor in the Department of Psychiatry at McGill University in Montreal, believes that the laying on of hands is an actual healing force. Because of a series of experiments which he conducted with healer Oskar Estebany in the 1950s, Dr. Grad believes that the healing effects of such energy are real and that further research might produce substantial medical benefits.

In a 1972 interview with Tom Harpur, religion editor of the Toronto *Star,* Dr. Grad said that he believes the religious rite of laying on of hands releases an actual force or energy that can be tested under laboratory conditions. In addition, the Montreal biologist is also convinced that an "unseen energy or vital force" is released in all forms of human contact, from a kiss to simply shaking hands.

"It's what every mother knows," Dr. Grad told Harpur. "You comfort a child by holding it. I believe it happens when food is blessed by grace . . . or when a woman prepares her cooking with love. What is new in my work is that we have shown this energy to be something real and verifiable. It is at its peak in healers. . . .

"My personal experience is that there are different qualities of healing energy. A personal element of the healer may go along with this power and if he himself is not moved by true selflessness and concern for others, the results could be negative . . . . The healer must be concerned about his own spiritual state and live a moral life."

Inspired by the work of Russian scientists with Kirlian photography, wherein objects display brightly colored coronas around their edges and the hands of healers appear to have extra wide coronas, Dr. Thelma Moss, a UCLA psychologist and Dr. Marshall Barshay, a Veterans Administration kidney specialist, investigated the powers of men and women who claim to cure illness by the "laying on of hands." Dr. Moss said in a recent interview that she strongly believed that the auras were "something which radiates from the body of a person with healing power."

The series of experiments which polygraph expert Cleve Backster has been conducting with plants is relevant to a discussion of healing, because the demonstrations of Backster Research Foundation imply that all life is one, that there is a signal linkage which exists among all living things, that there is unity to all creation. Such a belief is basic to medicine power, as well as to the essential tenets of all great metaphysicians and the inspired men and women of history. How wonderful if science's most sophisticated equipment might offer demonstrable proof of that ancient assertion.

Backster told the *Wall Street Journal* that in addition to giving evidence of a telepathic communication system, the plants monitored by his polygraphs also possess "something closely akin to feelings or emotions. . . . They appreciate being watered. They worry when a dog comes near. They faint when violence threatens their own well-being, and they sympathize when harm comes to animals and insects close to them."

On one occasion when Backster connected an egg to the polygraph, the recording showed the heartbeat of an embryo chick. Since the egg was a non-incubated, fresh egg with no physical circulatory system to account for the appropriate 170 beats per minute, Backster has theorized that there might be an "energy field blueprint" that provides a rhythm and pattern about which matter may coalesce to form organic structures.

In an article on Backster's work in *Psychic* magazine, John W. White asks: "Does the 'idea' of an organism precede its material development? Perhaps this is evidence for what the Bible and Plato say: In the beginning was the Logos—the structuring principle of the thought-form of the entity-to-be."

Dr. Harold Saxton Burr hypothesizes in his *Blueprint for Immortality* that man, animals, and vegetables have distinctive electrical field patterns. Since all protoplasmic systems have inherent electrodynamic fields and since every living system is composed of protoplasm (a reactive tissue) every organism thereby possesses the progenitor of a nervous system because it is also composed of protoplasm. Dr. Burr told John White that there was a universality to the electrodynamic field phenomena: "It's everywhere, all through the universe and all through you and me and plants—a field that can be measured by electrical instruments."

The electromagnetic vibrations given off by minerals such as quartz crystals have long been thought to have healing powers. Oh-Shinnah is a researcher and healer who shares her thoughts in the following interview which originally appeared in *Expansion* newsletter (July–August 1981) and is reprinted here by permission of the author, Caroline Myss.

Oh-Shinnah—a woman small in structure, powerful in spirit—says of herself, "I prefer to be known as one with no history and as a confrontation to fixed reality. We attach such importance to things like data, personal credentials. We get all caught up in that and never see the person.

"My blood is primarily Indian. My heart is of the earth," continued Oh-Shinnah. "I believe that knowledge and wisdom stand on their own volition."

And indeed, knowledge and wisdom seem to guide the abilities and thoughts of this woman, who is a trained psychologist, a Native American, a healer and a leading expert in the area of working with crystals. Oh-Shinnah uses her knowledge of crystals in her work as a healer and it has earned her the respect of both the scientific and medical communities.

"All of my work areas promote healing, and not necessarily always the healing of the body. Sometimes healing is allowing the body to cease and desist and allowing the spirit to go on," Oh-Shinnah said. "And I work with healing the planet because I really don't believe there is healing on any level until the planet itself is healed. What we are as human beings is reflected in our environment, and we're polluted."

Oh-Shinnah acquired her knowledge of crystals from, as she described it, two sides of the road. "My primary learning was from my great-grandmother, who was a Mohawk, and my father, who is full-blood Apache. I grew up with it. My great-grandmother gave me hers when she crossed over. I was eighteen. She said I could keep the crystal and that it was my key to get back and forth between her in this world and in the next. Crystals are magic. They really are. They'll come to you when it's time for you to have them," Oh-Shinnah said.

"I've learned about crystals from the Mayans, from the Navajo and from a Tibetan teacher. Apache people have always used them. Almost all native peoples everywhere in the world have used crystals. I wondered why and I started researching it. There is all sorts of scientific data that covers what is going on with crystals on the physical realm," Oh-Shinnah said.

"I believe that today's mysticism is tomorrow's science. And what we're doing is catching up linguistically to what is being done on spiritual levels. We already live in a crystal technology. The major component of watches is a crystal and in computers, the crystal is the memory bank. So that indicates to me that what my great-grandmother told me about being able to charge them—to program them—makes absolute sense. I can take a crystal and I can breathe my intentionality into it and program it to do a certain work for me.

"And the body, being 78 to 96 percent water, is a liquid crystal. If you examine the skin with a microscope, you will see little crystals, not to mention the blood and urine crystals," Oh-Shinnah stated.

"A small crystal set next to a very large crystal will come up and duplicate the electromagnetic vibration of the larger crystal. When you put a crystal on, it elevates all the little body crystals and they will duplicate the vibration of the larger crystal, or the one you're wearing. And coupling with your own electromagnetic field, the crystal increases your field energy in front of you. It's like a vortex of energy. They also have a refractive index. They push energy away," said Oh-Shinnah.

Oh-Shinnah emphasized that the most important point to remember about crystals is that they magnify intention. "I work primarily with quartz crystals. Clarity is very important in a crystal and you don't want to work with a real tiny one. I literally breathe into a crystal and while I'm doing that, I am thinking my intention. I am breathing my intention into the crystal. There is power in the breath," she said.

Oh-Shinnah said that before actually going to work on a patient, she does an assessment by moving the crystal through the person's electromagnetic field to find out what is in the field itself. "I counsel with them to find out if the problem they are dealing with is a current life problem, or a childhood problem or a past-life problem.

"I use everything in healing—color, therapeutic touch, tones—anything that works. The crystals work within the realms of sonics very, very well. They resonate with a tone. I believe I've figured out a way where I can recognize the tone in the crystals just by holding the crystals in my left hand, which stimulates activity in the right brain hemisphere, or the creative, intuitive process, and then listening and duplicating what I'm hearing in my head and singing that tone. I've learned to vibrate tones or frequencies that open the solar plexus and heart chakras so that healing energies can be taken in," Oh-Shinnah said.

"If I'm working with a cancer patient, I would breathe an intention into the crystal to help this person to heal. If the specific problem was cancer of the liver, and I've programmed the crystal to work specifically with those problems, sometimes I'll be working on the liver where the disease is and all of a sudden, the crystal is moving up to where the heart is. This tells me that the reason the person has cancer in the first place is because they are blocked in the heart chakra. So I start talking to them and sure enough, they are very blocked individuals," Oh-Shinnah continued. She also noted that crystals can be used to remove pain.

Oh-Shinnah has been doing workshops for many years. She estimates that she has trained forty thousand people, mostly nurses. Further, she believes that nurses will eventually change the entire medical profession, moving it toward a more holistic approach. Oh-Shinnah stated that it takes two to three three-day workshops to acquire a beginner's knowledge and ability in working with crystals, in addition to a good deal of practice.

Presently, Oh-Shinnah is involved in a research project with Dolores Krieger, Ph.D., director of the Ph.D. and Master's program at New York University School of Nursing and author of *Therapeutic Touch* and *Foundations for Holistic Health Nursing Practices.*

"Primarily, what I'm doing with Dee is research on what is going on with natural quartz crystals and therapeutic touch because we've had some results that we don't understand—one of them was the day we found out that it works," Oh-Shinnah said. "You see, one of the reasons the medical community listens to me is because of results. I don't have a great deal of research yet on how or why it works, but they've already seen that it does work.

"Dee and I were doing a workshop in California. It was around Easter time and this particular little girl and her father were coloring Easter eggs.

She and her father had a fight and she pulled the pot of boiling water over on herself and received third-degree burns on her legs. They took her to the hospital and shot her up with Demerol. They said she would not even be able to be on her legs for three weeks and that healing would not set in for a long time. She was still in agony when they brought her to us," continued Oh-Shinnah.

"Dee immediately started doing Therapeutic Touch and I started working in the same area with the crystal. All of a sudden, I felt the crystal tugging at me and I realized it was heading toward the solar plexus. I realized that what happened was that in her anger, she pulled the water over herself and tightened up her solar plexus (stomach area) so that the energy of fear and shock were contained in that area and that she was holding it there and not in her legs. So I started working in that area and as I did, Dee starting getting discharges of energy into her hands so fast that she had to call in another nurse trained in Therapeutic Touch to help ground her. There were thirty people standing around us and we literally watched all the red peripheral areas start to move in and shrink, all of the blisters infiltrated and then, very slowly, this kind of filmy substance went over the third degree burn area. That little girl was on her bicycle the next day and was free from pain from that moment on," Oh-Shinnah said.

"So we started saying, hey, something is going on here. The crystal, being a magnifier, would magnify the intention of Therapeutic Touch in addition to its own healing properties. Therapeutic Touch elevates the hemoglobin and changes the enzyme system. Dee and I are going to try to replicate these experiments to see if there isn't some way we can test what happens with a patient, first with just Therapeutic Touch and then with Therapeutic Touch and the crystals. We're looking to find out if healing increases using both techniques. This will probably be done at New York University," Oh-Shinnah said.

While Oh-Shinnah insists that anyone can be taught to use a crystal, she stated, "It is in our tradition that crystal should be given to you. To allow a crystal to come to you is an indication from other energies that it's time. I think the Western world is in a very big hurry. I call it spiritual materialism. Everybody wants it all now; they don't perfect anything they learn. They learn a little about something and they do tremendous damage because they are not experts. The Western world thinks they can go out and buy everything. They are all looking for miracles to happen in their lives and they ignore the little miracles, like maybe just developing enough patience to allow things to be given to you. Buying a crystal programs it immediately with the attitude that I can buy whatever I want."

Oh-Shinnah added that it is possible for a person to buy his/her own crystal in the event that one is not given to them. These can be worn for protection and for heightening one's own energy field. The crystal used in healing, however, should be one given to an individual.

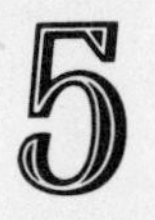

"Black Robes" and the Old Traditions

> Morley, Alberta, August 19, 1972—When the Reverend John S. Hascall, an American Roman Catholic priest, says mass he prefers a teepee to a church.
>
> Several nights ago he sat crosslegged on the ground in a large white teepee illuminated by a campfire of poplar logs. His vestments were not white but black, the traditional sacred color of American Indians, and the Lord's Prayer was in Cree.
>
> In his homily he spoke of Jesus Christ as a "Holy Man" sent to put men in contact with the Great Spirit.
>
> Father Hascall is an Ojibwa Indian, and like a growing number of members of his race—some Christian and some not—he has committed himself to the revival of native religious traditions.
>
> This weekend, Father Hascall and more than 600 other Indians of similar persuasion gathered on the Stoney Indian Reserve in the foothills of the Canadian Rockies for the third annual Indian Ecumenical Conference. The conference underscored the growing interest among Indians in their religious heritage. [Edward B. Fiske, special to the *New York Times*]

When I contacted Father Hascall, a Franciscan Capuchin of the province of St. Joseph, a priest of an all-Indian parish in Baraga, Michigan, he was in the midst of plastering a wall in his parish house. I apologized and offered to call again at a more convenient time, but Father Hascall said he would be happy to take a cigarette break and answer my questions.

Why do you believe that American Indians are beginning to commit themselves to a revival of native religious traditions at this time?

Father Hascall: "What happened is this: We have our medicine men, our holy men; we look in the past and we see the future; we look at the future and see the present. And we find that Christianity has been here since 1492 and it has not yet caught on with our people. There must be something wrong.

"We had a very religious people before the whiteman came. Now our children are disobeying their parents; they are committing suicide; they are doing all kinds of evil things which they never did before when we had our own religion. Let me say, if this is the way Christianity is going to be, we will have to go back to our old ways."

Do you feel that the religious traditions of Europe or Asia can be compatible with Native American religious traditions?

Father Hascall: "If you mean European traditions with European rites, no. If you mean the Christian religion as Christ taught it, yes. I know both religions, and I see nothing incompatible.

"The essential message of Christ was love. Love has always been in our people. But a lot of the dogma can be irrelevant."

Are you going to retain your status in the Roman Catholic Church?

Father Hascall: "Yes, I will always be a priest. I will always be a Christian, an Indian Christian. Our two ways are compatible as religion, but not as rite."

How would you prefer to conduct mass in accordance with Indian tradition?

Father Hascall: "Mass wouldn't be celebrated every week. I would schedule big days of celebration. Within those days, I would serve the Eucharist."

You would make it a true agape, or love feast, then?

Father Hascall: "Right, as it was in the early days of the Christian Church."

It seems to me that you are talking about the possibility of blending Apostolic Christianity with the native traditions of your people.

Father Hascall: "Right, Apostolic Christianity as it was in the first century, or so. This is the true Christianity. There was not the bureaucracy that we have now.

"I would say that now we are seeing the Holy Spirit bringing more relevance to the kind of nature religion that is the Indian way. This religion of the Spirit moving and working in all things was born in this country. It is the religion the Spirit gave to this country. We know that we have only one God and that His Spirit works in all creatures and all things, even the stones.

"The Indian has his rites—the puberty rites, the marriage rites, the death rites. The Indian has a priesthood. I want to be able to see the Christian Church come forth and blend with the way our people have been doing things for thirty thousand years. The Lateran Council has recommended such action in other countries, but our bishop and our Church won't allow us to do it here."

Do you in your personal life utilize dreams and visions?

Father Hascall: "Yes, I use medicine myself. I follow both religions."

Do you have any particular techniques for inducing dreams and visions?

Father Hascall: "I would say it is through contemplation. He will speak when He wants to speak. It is not something I force. Twenty-five years ago, the young men of my tribe would go out and find our totem, our spirit vision. I never did it myself, though."

How do you deal with the Roman Catholic tradition of saints?

Father Hascall: "I would say saints are our elders. There are always holy people in the tribes. The saints are our grandmothers and grandfathers who are in spirit and who yet pray with us in our church."

Can American Indian traditions offer a workable faith for today?

Father Hascall: "I would say so for the Indians. The white people have their religion. As a whole, I do not think it is possible for a whiteman to adapt himself easily to the native traditions.

"I do believe, though, that Apostolic Christianity, wherein one's faith becomes a total part of his lifestyle, can be made compatible with native American traditions. That is why I can be a priest. I know if the Spirit has led me this far, He has a reason for it."

Can Christianity, the religion that Manifest Destiny seized upon and distorted to help win the West, really be made compatible with the spiritual traditions of the American Indians?

The Native Americans, together with other minority groups, have noted the effort on the part of church leaders to make Christianity relevant by depicting "black Christs" and by distributing Christmas cards portraying the Holy Family living in a hogan on the Navajo reservation. Vine Deloria, Jr., finds such attempts to transpose the Christian mythos and archetypes into Indian, black, and Mexican terms to be "totally patronizing and unrealistic." In *We Talk, You Listen,* he writes:

> This type of religious paternalism overlooks the fact that the original figures of religious myths were designed to communicate doctrines. It satisfies itself by presenting its basic figures as so

> universalized that anyone can participate at any time in history. Thus the religion that it is trying to communicate becomes ahistorical, as Mickey Mouse and Snow White are ahistorical.

As I talked to a number of Native Americans, I found there were differences of opinion as to how much harm or good the "Black Robes" (the Christian missionaries) had done to the early Indian and as to how well Christianity and the old traditions might blend.

Twylah, Seneca: "Do I feel the religious traditions of Christianity can be compatible with Native American traditions? No. No way.

"Now first of all, I must tell you that my great-grandfather was an early convert to Christianity, and, in fact, he became a minister as well as a teacher. His name was Daniel Webster Pierce, and he was the man who built the house in which I was born on the reservation.

"When the French missionaries introduced Christianity to our people, there were four main reasons the Senecas found it difficult to embrace the faith:

"First, Christianity is a religion, a system of faith and worship. It appeared to the Indian that the followers of Christianity donned their religion only when the need arose. They spoke of beautiful philosophy and spent entire days in prayer, but, the following day, all these things lost their meaning, whereas Indian faith and worship was a daily lifestyle.

"Second, Christianity seemed to be a religion of supplication, whereas, Indian thoughts were praises of thanksgiving. Christianity did not provide a place for the Indians to conduct their expressions of thanksgiving, which were customarily carried out in ceremonials of song, dance, and feasts (Condolences, Green Corn Dances, etc.).

"Third, Christianity introduced only one 'Earthwalk' with souls waiting for the return of Christ for resurrection. Indians believed in experiencing many former lives that provided countless lessons during each earth visit. These evolutionary experiences did not have to be repeated, because, after their completion, the spirited energy (soul) returned to the Happy Hunting Ground to await the next environmental lessons that would ultimately lead to eternal peace. Creatures are now evolving in the Fourth World.

"And fourth, our teachers told us about *Swenio,* the Great Mystery that in latter days became known as the Great Spirit. This spiritual essence resides in every manifestation in the universe and is present at all times, everywhere for time eternal. This spiritual essence is not a male image dwelling somewhere in outer space. To us, everything seen or unseen, throughout our awareness, is an image of the Creator (God), and there is only one. We are made from this same Spirit substance; therefore, all things are related—the plants, animals, birds, stone—you name it, and we are all kin.

"In the mind of the Indian, Christianity limited the magnificent gifts and powers of our Creator. Jesus Christ had evolved to a high dimension of spirituality and taught these loving principles for others to emulate. This is the reason some Indians embraced Christianity.

"Because of this Great Spirit substance endowed by the Creator to earthlings, there was no need to have priests or others to handle our transgressions. We were told that these were our responsibilities. All our lessons were to help us learn the ways of living in harmony within our environment. Since these lessons were to be learned and assessed according to our gifts and abilities as we walked our daily path of life, our happiness (heaven) or discomfort (hell) was here and now. We did not have to pay for mistakes handed down from a former life. At death, the lessons of this particular earth experience had been fulfilled. Those who did not have this instruction often became drifters on their way to the Happy Hunting Ground and were often helped by sensitive people who performed releasing ceremonies.

"In short, converts embraced Christianity because they loved the life of Jesus Christ who taught such good medicine. Some people defined their belief as interchangeable—Lord and Great Spirit. I do and so did my family.

"We could not understand why there had to be so much blood shed in the name of religion. Our Creator is not an angry God. Only loving, healing, and righteousness are present with every breath we take. Never are we alone with this belief. It only appears to others that we walk alone.

"I am aware of my former lives, or forms of evolution, because they are my source of spiritual and material seeking. My Clan is the Wolf, preceded by the Deer. There is a lesson for me in this identity. I have lived wolf and deer lifestyles (family characteristics, instincts). Therefore, in each of my former life experiences, I carry this knowledge crystallized in my present personality.

" 'There would be no growth without the framework of former lives to support the present life.' How often these words have been spoken by medicine teachers and people of wisdom.

"We are born into this physical environment to experience growing in a family of our choice and Nature's universal family.

"We have talents, qualities of character, and abilities that have been previously developed during former lives to assist us in preparing for the life that follows.

"In this life, our teachers are from spiritual dimensions of more advanced evolutions, as well as from those found in this physical environment.

"We have a mission in this life and will remain here until this mission is fulfilled. If we know what this mission is, we will understand the purpose for the discomforts we experience during this Earthwalk and will praise the Great Spirit for the lessons."

Dallas Chief Eagle, Sioux: "All religions are good. Perhaps, as in music, we progress best by achieving combinations.

"You know, Tchaikovsky's music was never appreciated until he combined German music with Russian. Puccini wasn't appreciated until he combined oriental music with Italian. Music is the simplest language in the world, understood by everyone.

"Maybe with a combination of different beliefs, we may accommodate each other so that we do not destroy each other. The greatest gift Christ gave in his teachings was the element of love. I think this is one of the greatest gaps that Christianity has overlooked—the lifestyle of Christ. It is this same element of love that the Indians have in their belief in the 'humanhood.' "

Sun Bear, Chippewa: "I feel the two traditions are incompatible. I feel that the medicine of the European Christians is for their continent. I think that many of the visions and prophecies of our people are for our people here.

"I don't feel we need to argue about these things. If I say my ancestor was a bear and you say your ancestor was a monkey, we don't have to fight, you know. We don't have to kill each other or pour lead in each other's ears to bring about conversions. That is not the Indian way."

Rarihokwats, Mohawk: "Indians have always been a great people not to make hasty judgments and to let things go their course. If they don't like something, they withdraw from it, rather than confront it. I think that the Indians have resisted to a high degree by nonparticipation. Indians are masterful nonparticipants.

"I think that although there are many Indians who are devout Christians, there are many others who have dabbled in Christianity and have found it seriously lacking.

"I think, more than anything, Indians right now are at a stage of history when they are saying: 'Okay, we tried Christianity and it doesn't work. We can see what has happened with a Christian nation as it flowered. We now know what the flower smells like, and we just don't like it. We have decided that we don't like the sample. We are not going to participate any further.'

"The problem that many contemporary Indians face is that they have gone through white semi-military boarding school situations. They have accepted the Indian stereotype that non-Indians have and, in many ways, become very white in their thought patterns. They have accepted the Indian stereotype that non-Indians have foisted upon them. They think that they already are Indian and all they have to do is to find the nearest medicine man, let him do some kind of thing, and they will instantly be back into the tradition. Of course many of them become impatient when they find that the medicine people are not terribly enthusiastic. The medicine people are very hospitable, and so on, but they just are not able to give these people the instant religion for which they are looking.

"You can become an instant Christian, but you can't become an instant Indian.

"I am not going to criticize other people who say that they are both Christian and Indian, because, apparently, in some way, they have been able to make that synthesis. I can't, because I find too many incompatible elements that I am not able to live with.

"I think there are now more Christian Indians who are able to find elements of Indian religion satisfying who are coming back to their Indian-ness, than there are practitioners of Indian religion who head toward Christianity. I think these people who are fully in the Indian religion need nothing else. They don't want anything else. They are quite satisfied emotionally and every other way, and there is no need for them to turn to Christianity. But Christians now are lacking in something, and they are turning to Indian religion to get what they are missing.

"I think another problem that Western people have is their concept of time as being some sort of a progression. There are many religious beliefs which are not caught into that kind of time, beliefs that are universal and present in every era. There is really no such thing as becoming 'modern' with these beliefs. They are good anytime.

"The thing that Christians generally forget is that their own religion goes back two thousand years, and on the Judeo aspect, a great deal longer than that. Yet Christians somehow see themselves as holding *the* modern religion, while the Indian religion is old-fashioned and outdated. I just don't think that most Christians understand their own religious beliefs that well."

In a special report to the *New York Times,* Edward B. Fiske quoted John Snow, a chief of the Stony tribe, who hosted the third annual Indian Ecumenical Conference: "Our people are beginning to realize that we have a religious faith that is as good as any other. After many years of seeing it condemned as pagan—and accepting such judgments ourselves—we are ready again to take pride in it."

Wilfred Pelletier, a consultant to the Nishnawbe Institute, told Fiske: "Eating a meal, smoking a cigarette—these acts are all ceremonies to me. We are inseparable from the earth and the universe."

Earnest Tootoosis, a Plains Cree from Saskatchewan, and a delegate to the conference, remarked to the assembly: "We were in a Garden of Eden when the white man came in 1492, but now we have been destroyed. We must go back to the way our forefathers worshipped. We must pray to the Great Spirit the way he wanted us to."

Robert Thomas, a Cherokee who had helped organize the ecumenical conferences, noted that the Indian people were searching for some kind of structure and identity, and he speculated that such a search ". . . may end up creating a new Indian religion."

Reverend Andrew Ahendkew, a Plains Cree who is an Anglican, looks for a greater integration of Christian and Native American religious traditions. Although he admitted that he would like to go back to tribal tradition "100 percent," Reverend Ahendkew said that he could not. In his view Christianity and the old traditions "must live in harmony."

Is it possible for the old traditions of the Native Americans, with their emphasis on the individual's totality with the earth and the universe, to be harmonious with Christianity, which traditionally represents humans as having a sinful nature, yet, at the same time, authorizes them to have dominion over nature?

In *American Indian Religions,* John Major Hurdy writes:

> Christianity claims God's laws to be above natural law, not to be its sum total. Christianity has a history of obstructing the study of nature and suppressing information about nature. It represents man's nature as sinful and this planet in its beauty as being no more than a prison house to which our parents and their progeny have been condemned. It claims sorrow and retribution for our heritage and says that life itself is unimportant except as a path to heaven. . . .

> . . . [the Indians] were all oriented to the rhythm of creation. Without telescopes, the Indian visionaries felt the universe about them and dedicated themselves to keeping man's world in balance with the cosmos. All of them loved the earth and held her body and her children sacred. All of them sought to communicate with the powers of nature. Cumulatively they developed a variety of techniques for doing so. And [their religious traditions] were an integral part of the lives of the people. . . .

Dr. Walter Houston Clark, professor emeritus at Andover Newton Theological Seminary, agrees with Reverend Ahendkew about the harmonious future which Christianity and the traditional Indian beliefs might share.

Dr. Clark: "I noted that the peyote ceremony which I attended with the Potawatomi in Kansas was a syncretic one, which involved both Christian and traditional Indian elements. Personally, this was a congenial factor for me, being Christian in my general approach.

"I think that as we look at the history of religion, we see that this syncretism goes on all the time. Whenever there are two religious traditions close to one another, there is a tendency for the two traditions to draw nearer together, even though one of the traditions may be dominant. Certainly the Christian communion service, the mass, and so on, owe a great deal to many of the Eastern and Near Eastern mystery cults of two thousand or more years ago; and I see no reason why this shouldn't be the case today.

"For example, the peyote ceremony in which I participated was the most impressive religious ceremony that I have ever attended. For me, it would be an easy step toward using these drugs, or similar ones, under proper supervision.

"The supervision provided by the Indians in this service was superb. The man who was in charge was experienced, and the whole ceremony directed the experiences of the worshipers at that service. I see no reason why that kind of religious expertise couldn't be developed among the whites.

"When you get right down to the essential elements of religious life, as William James said, I think they are rooted in the mystical experiences of the individual. One of the characteristics of these drugs is their agency of releasing the mystical potentialities of men, no matter what they are.

"With this as groundwork, I think that almost any tradition could be linked with another tradition. It is when you get to the more superficial aspects of religious beliefs—the dogmas and self-righteous traditions—that you get into trouble.

"I think the American Indians' concern with Nature and the environment that surrounds them is another way in which one can open up the mystical core of his nature. In this respect, I think that the two traditions are compatible, at least to some degree."

In a speech at the University of Nebraska, a Chippewa named Bellecourt commented that American Indians were not against the concept of Christianity, but they were against the way it had been used against the Indian people. "Christianity was taught to the Indian by persons who broke all Ten Commandments," he said.

"Early in the history of North American exploration," Vine Deloria, Jr., has observed, "the fundamental responsibilities of Genesis became interpreted as man's right, and basically the whiteman's right, to use whatever he wanted and however he wanted to use it. Wholesale destruction of the forests, the game, and the original peoples of this continent were justified as part of God's plan to subdue and dominate an untamed wilderness. Nowhere was there any sense of stewardship between diverse elements of the new Christian settlers either collectively or individually and the continent as they found it. . . ."

M. Edward McGaa, a Sioux and assistant director of Minnesota Indian Education, remarked in a speech made at Navajo Community College's American Indian Seminar Series that Christian missionaries should stay off the reservations and devote more time to their own people.

"The white man's religion has destroyed our unity," McGaa said. "The white man's religion has no power. Yes, I believe in Christ. I believe he appeared to those people over there across the sea. He didn't appear to the Indians. All the tribes of North America have one God, the Great Spirit. We all have the same prophecies. All the things that are happening now were predicted.

"Indians don't argue religion; they don't try to force it on someone else. The white man does. . . . We've got to get back to our values, to our religion. We must spread our values to the world. Otherwise those people are going to blow each other up and some of us with them."

Although a number of white judges have ruled recently that young Indian men may receive conscientious objector status as a result of their ascribing to the traditional beliefs of their tribe, the vast majority of non-Indian citizens of the United States would probably show as much respect toward practitioners of medicine and tribal religious traditions as they would toward exponents of the flat earth society. At best, Native American medicine is regarded as quaint superstition and surviving bits of folklore. In order for the average non-Indian to consider treating medicine and the traditional American Indian beliefs seriously, s/he must come to terms with centuries of European heritage; and s/he must work out some kind of intellectual compromise with an educational background that has conditioned him or her to believe that *modern* and *technological* is good, and that *traditional* and *non-industrial* is bad.

To the Taos Indians of New Mexico, the watershed of the Sangre de Cristo Mountains is a natural temple of meditation. They grow no crops there. They do not harvest the trees for lumber. They are not interested in the possibility of any valuable minerals existing in the rocks. They have been making pilgrimages to Blue Lake for more than seven hundred years.

In July 1970, the Taos people came under challenge and ridicule by United States senators who saw no reason why the Taos Pueblo should have total control of 48,000 acres of timberland. It seemed unfathomable to the questioning senators that the Taos could hold a site so spiritual that they could resist the obvious financial advantage in exploiting the area.

What kind of real religion could it be that would consider trees, flowers, grass, rocks, and soil to be sacred? These things are for the two-leggeds, the apex of God's creation, to make use of as they will.

Former President Richard Nixon endorsed the Taos's request after meeting with their delegation and with the president of the National Congress of American Indians. In his prepared statement former President Nixon said:

> . . . From the fourteenth century, the Taos Pueblo Indians used these areas for religious and tribal purposes. In 1906, however, the United States government appropriated these lands for the creation of a national forest. According to a recent determination of the Indian Claims Commission, the government 'took said lands from petitioner without compensation.'
>
> For sixty-four years, the Taos Pueblo has been trying to regain possession of this sacred lake and watershed area in order to preserve its natural condition and limit its non-Indian use. The Taos Indians consider such action essential to the protection and expression of their religious faith. . . .

Senator Lee Metcalf of Montana worried about the danger of "medicine men springing up all over the country and asking for the same deal."

Quentin Burdick, senator from North Dakota, asked if Taos Pueblo would agree to a "reverter clause" to return the land to the United States Government in the event that the Taos would cease utilizing it for religious purposes. Maybe, Senator Burdick speculated, the Taos might change their minds and decide to go into the lumber and mining business.

Paul J. Bernal, secretary of the Pueblo Council, indignantly retorted that it was apparent that the senators did not believe the Taos's explanation of their religion.

"We are not accepting any reverter," Bernal told the interior subcommittee. "We are not going to use this land for anything but religion. We are going to give this land back to nobody."

Former Interior Secretary Walter Hickel threw his lot in with the Taos, stating that while his department would not look with favor on every request of such nature, the Taos Pueblo situation was "unique" because of the established record of their having petitioned for the return of their shrine for sixty-four years.

"The administration will take a different stand for religious reasons than economic," former Secretary Hickel said.

Orthodox white religions have little difficulty obtaining tax-exempt status. They may send letters of solicitation through the mails, and they may acquire land holdings and market investments, while remaining secure in their "nonprofit organization" seal. The Taos Pueblo had to petition for sixty-four years in order to convince the United States Government that they should be permitted to achieve total control of a site that had been the focal point of sacred pilgrimages for seven hundred years.

It would be difficult to conceive of a Senate subcommittee convening to challenge bishops and cardinals on the matter of tax exemption on the wealth and financial holdings of the Roman Catholic Church. But think of all the tax revenue the government is losing because the Taos have these superstitions regarding 48,000 acres of rich timberland and potentially rich mineral deposits! Why, if this were one hundred years ago, we could easily pass the proper legislation or break the appropriate treaty and see to it that the watershed of the Sangre de Cristo would be correctly developed. We certainly would not permit ridiculous native beliefs about the sacredness of an area to stop us. How pagan. How downright pantheistic. Trees, mountains, and lakes are not sacred. Cathedrals, churches, and synagogues are sacred. Maybe all these bleeding hearts in the country have made us too damn soft.

In regard to the exploitation of natural resources and the "justification" of disregarding native traditions that might inhibit the commercial development of the Earth Mother, Vine Deloria, Jr. had an appropriate answer to this ridiculous and all too familiar kind of reasoning. In "An Open Letter to the Heads of the Christian Churches," he said:

> The poverty we presently endure, the confiscation of our lands, the destruction of animals we once enjoyed, the obliteration of our valleys and rivers, the exploitation of our holy places as tourist traps, all of these things might have occurred anyway. We might even have done these things eventually, although according to our beliefs this would have been the gravest of sins.
>
> But we would never have deliberately done these things as a religious command. . . .
>
> It may be that we cannot change the past, but we can certainly begin to try to understand it. We have only to stand today for the things that are right, and which we know are right. If promises have been made, those promises must be kept. If mistakes are made, they must be corrected. If the lands of aboriginal peoples were wrongly taken by a Christian mandate, then what remains of those lands must not be continually taken once the mistake is known.
>
> It remains to you as honest men to ponder what your predecessors have created, and what, by your silence, you now endorse. . . . You must renounce the errors that have led men astray from themselves, and lead the search for that understanding or that religious interpretation that can bring them to understand themselves, their fellow men, and the creation in which they live. . . .
>
> *O Great Spirit, grant us understanding!*

One cannot doubt the sincerity of the early Christian missionaries, the Black Robes, who earnestly attempted to preach what they considered the authentic word of God to the American Indians. However, understanding between peoples is all but impossible if one people regard their culture, their customs, and their religion as innately superior, and all discourse is intoned in a paternal and patronizing manner.

"Lost in the dark the heathen doth languish," bemoans a familiar missionary hymn, soundly implying that there is a single source of illumination. When the Black Robes set forth on their spiritual safaris intent upon bringing light to the lost children of nature, they comfortably established themselves in the parental role and widened the gap of understanding between religious traditions.

In 1824 Chief Red Jacket of the Senecas clearly set forth his objections to the Christian missionaries:

> . . . [the missionaries] know we do not understand their religion. We cannot read their book—they tell us different stories about what it contains, and we believe they make the book talk to suit themselves. If we had no money, no land . . . to be cheated out of these black coats would not trouble themselves about our good hereafter.
>
> The Great Spirit will not punish us for what we do not know. He will do justice to his red children. These black coats talk to the Great Spirit, and ask for light that we may see as they do, when they are blind themselves and quarrel about the light that guides them. These things we do not understand, and the light which they give us makes the straight and plain path trod by our fathers dark and dreary.
>
> The black coats tell us to work and raise corn; they do nothing themselves and would starve to death if someone did not feed them. All they do is pray to the Great Spirit; but that will not make corn and potatoes grow; if it will why do they beg from us and from the white people? . . . As soon as they crossed the great waters they wanted our country, and in return have always been ready to teach us to quarrel about their religion. . . . If [the Indians] were raised among white people, and learned to work and read as they do, it would only make their situation worse. . . . We are few and weak, but may for a long time be happy if we hold fast to our country and the religion of our fathers.

The Black Coats, good Christian soldiers, marched onward to war against the redman's resolve to hold fast to the religion of his fathers. The missionaries had a divine crusade to save the Indians' souls. To leave them wallowing like animals in their pagan beliefs would have been unthinkable, an affront to the Apostolic commission to spread the word to the uttermost parts of the earth. The salvation of the Indian was but another weight to be added to the whiteman's burden, a weight to be shouldered willingly, since, of all races, the white had designated itself to be the keeper of its brothers.

Any number of missionaries might have forearmed themselves during their seminary training by reading *Information Respecting the History, Condition and Prospects of the Indian Tribes of the United States: Collected and Prepared Under the Direction of the Bureau of Indian Affairs, per Act of Congress of March 3d, 1847,* by Henry R. Schoolcraft, LL.D. In one of the papers collected therein, Lieutenant U.S.N. George Falconer Emmons characterizes the Indian in the following manner:

> Finally, as a race, although they differ materially in language, in point of mental and physical development, and the color of their hair, eyes, and skin, I question if they differ more from each other

> than the people occupying the extremes of the United States. They are generally well formed, below the whites in stature, have an easy gait, but neither graceful nor handsome; their eyes and hair usually black—the latter occasionally brown, generally parted in the middle of the forehead, so as to hang down each side; noses broad and flat—some aquiline exceptions. The mouth large, lips thick, teeth fair, but in adults generally more or less worn.

Once the seminarian had formed a mental image of his future children-of-nature parishioners as squat, ugly, clumsy, black-eyed people with worn teeth, he was presented with a summation of their character:

> They are wily, superstitious, lazy, indolent, and dirty. With these traits, united to an implacable hostility which they generally entertain towards the whites, it does not, I think, require much wisdom to predict their fate. [At this point, Manifest Destiny seemed to be placing a limit on the length of time the Indian salvation game could be played. There would be a reduced number of Indian souls for each missionary to save.]
>
> Facts that have developed themselves within the last year relating to these tribes, must, I think, convince the observing that Indian agencies and treaties cannot alone save them. It is melancholy to see them melting away so rapidly; but it does not appear to be intended that civilization should prevent it.

In another paper included in the report, Philander Prescott, United States Dacotah Interpreter from the Fort Snelling Agency in Minnesota, answered such specific questions about the religious life of the American Indians as the following:

> "What species or degree of worship do they, *in fine*, render to the Great Spirit? Do they praise him in hymns, chants, or choruses? Do they pray to him, and if so, for what purpose?"
>
> To analyze the worship of Indians, in our view, amounts to nothing at all. They are very tenacious and say they are right, and are very zealous and cling to their old habits like death, and will not give way to any kind of teaching. They pray, but their prayers are very short. . . .
>
> "Is there reason to believe the Indians to be idolators? Are images of wood or stone ever worshipped? . . . or is there any gross and palpable form of idolatry in the existing tribes, similar to that of the oriental world?"
>
> The Dacotahs have no images of wood that they worship, nor have they any edifices for public worship. These Indians worship in their natural state. An Indian will pick up a round stone, of any kind, and paint it, and go a few rods from his lodge, and clean away the grass, say from one to two feet in diameter, and there place his

> stone, or god, as he would term it, and make an offering of some tobacco and some feathers, and pray to the stone to deliver him from some danger that he has probably dreamed of, or from imagination.
>
> "Do they believe in the immortality of the soul, and the doctrine of moral accountability to the Creator? Do they believe in the resurrection of the body? Do they believe, at all, in the doctrine of reward and punishments in a future state?"
>
> The Indians believe in the immortality of the soul, but as for accountability they have but a vague idea of it. Future rewards and punishments they have no conception of. . . . Everything appears to be dark and mysterious with them respecting the future state of both the soul and the body.

When J. Lee Humfreville published his *Twenty Years Among Our Hostile Indians* in 1899, the authorities on Native American life who had actually lived among many tribes—without truly understanding any of them—were already referring to the aboriginal peoples in the past tense. However, the seminarian of that generation might well have added a book such as Humfreville's to his reading list, along with Bureau of Indian Affairs reports, so that he might save what few souls remained on the reservations. Even a casual perusal of *Twenty Years Among Our Hostile Indians* would cause the Christian soldier to gird his loins for a bitter fight with Satan among the redmen. Among his observations, Humfreville included these analyses:

> [The Indian] depended upon his natural animal instinct more than on human judgment. Yet, granting his superiority in these and other ways, he could not compete with civilized man.
>
> There was in the Indian nature a trait of intractability not found in any other portion of the human race. . . . He could not be enslaved. The Spaniards in the early days of discovery endeavored to enslave the Indian; the result was that he died in his chains. He was the same when I first knew him as he was then—unamenable to the law and impatient of restraint. . . . He might be brought up in the midst of civilized surroundings and educated, but at the first opportunity he would relapse into his original barbarism. . . .
>
> He was the very impersonation of duplicity. He might enter the cabin of a frontiersman, or a military fort, or an Indian agency, and listen to all that was said, without giving the slightest evidence that he understood what he heard, or that he was taking notice of his surroundings. In his attitude and facial expressions, he might appear as taciturn as a Sphynx, and yet understand every word that was uttered and be planning a murderous raid at the same moment.
>
> Occasionally, it is true, the Indian evinced some commendable traits of character. But these were the exception to the rule.

> Doubtless there are also instances of truthfulness and fidelity on his part. But granting this, it is still an indisputable fact that the Indian, of all uncivilized people, has offered the greatest degree of opposition to the influences of civilization.

In spite of the fact that the fledgling Black Coat was forewarned that the American Indian was ugly, clumsy, lazy, dirty, superstitious, deceitful, untruthful, and stubbornly opposed to being either enslaved or civilized, the Christian Light Bearers discovered many elements within American Indian tradition which they were hard put to explain. How, for example, had these primitive, isolated savages come to know so many of the Old Testament stories which the eager missionaries believed they were revealing to the pagan children of nature for the first time?

The Delaware, for example, told the stories of the Creation and the Great Deluge in pictographs that their people who were wise in the old traditions translated for the Black Coats. From a translation obtained by Professor C.S. Rafinesque in 1822, paraphrased in *Indian Myths,* Ellen Russell Emerson, 1884:

THE CREATION

At the first there were great waters above all land,
And above the waters were thick clouds, and there was God the Creator.
The first being, eternal, omnipotent, invisible, was God the Creator.
He created the sun, the moon, and stars.
He caused them all to move well.
By his power he made the winds to blow, purifying, and the deep waters to run off.
All was made bright, and the islands were brought into being.
Then again God the Creator made the great spirits.
He made also the first beings, guardians, and souls.
Then he made a man being, the father of man.
He gave him the first mother, the mother of the early born.
Fishes gave he him, turtles, beasts, and birds.
But the Evil Spirit created evil beings, snakes and monsters.
He created vermin and annoying insects.
Then were all beings friends.
There being a good god, all spirits were good—
The beings, the first men, mothers, wives, little spirits also.
Fat fruits were the food of the beings and the little spirits.
All were then happy, easy in mind, and pleased.
But then came secretly on earth the snake god, the snake-priest, and snake-worship.
Came wickedness, came unhappiness.
Came then bad weather, disease, and death.
This was all very long ago, at our early home.

THE GREAT DELUGE

Long ago came the powerful serpent, when men had become evil.
The strong serpent was the foe of the beings; and they became embroiled, hating each other.
Then they fought and despoiled each other, and were not peaceful.
And the small men fought with the keeper of the dead.
Then the strong serpent resolved all men and beings to destroy immediately.
The black serpent monster brought the snake-water rushing.
The wide waters rushing wide to the hills, everywhere spreading, everywhere destroying.
At the island of the turtle was Manabozho, of men and beings the Grand-father.
Being born creeping, at turtle-land he is ready to move and dwell.
Men and beings go forth on the flood of waters, moving afloat every way, seeking the back of the turtle.
The monsters of the sea were many, and destroyed some of them.
Then the daughter of a spirit helped them in a boat, and all joined saying, Come, help!
Manabozho, of all beings, of men and turtles, the Grand-father!
All together, on the turtle then, the men then, were all together.
Much frightened, Manabozho prayed to the turtle that he would make all well again.
Then the waters ran off, it was dry on mountain and plain, and the great evil went elsewhere by the path of the cave.

Tribe after tribe across the length and width of the continent had legends and myths which closely paralleled the accounts found in Genesis and in other books of the Old Testament. Some missionaries dealt with the problem in the same manner that the early Spanish priests had dealt with the Aztec myths: they declared that the native peoples had been told these stories by Satan.

In his study of the aboriginal peoples written during the last century, an indignant John Tanner fulminated against such accounts related by the medicine men and declared: "If the Great Spirit had communications to make, he would make them through a *white* man, not an Indian!"

Other Christian scholars and missionaries were not so certain, and a theory which held that the aboriginal peoples were the descendants of the Lost Tribes of Israel was formulated in an effort to explain the similarity between so many of the Indians' legends, rites, and word sounds and Israeli counterparts. To add a kind of intriguing credence to this theory was the enigma of the Mandan tribe—blue-eyed, fair-complexioned native peoples of the central plains. Clergymen set out with renewed vigor in an effort to reclaim the scattered Israeli tribes, lost to the fold for so long, denied the opportunity to accept Jesus as the Messiah, and condemned to wander a pagan land with their holy traditions but dim memories.

Most of the early scholars, and it appears the majority of secular and clerical authorities, today hold fast to the explanation of acculturation and the idea that the early Indians borrowed and adapted the Christian cosmology in terms of their own environment. Even in our liberal times, too many authorities see the Native American as spiritually retarded at the time of the whiteman's advent to this continent. At best, the aboriginal peoples are seen as superstitious, pantheistic children of nature who prayed to every clap of thunder and every shaking bush.

"As a result of such attitudes, we have gone underground in many things," Don Wilkerson of the Arizona Indian Centers in Phoenix told me.

Don Wilkerson: "The missionary influence has, in many respects, caused the Indian religions and the Indian beliefs to withdraw from their view. No one likes to be laughed at, and no one likes to be humiliated.

"As far as our not having any culture or religion, I can point to the Hopi, whose religious traditions go back thousands of years. Their ancient prophecies are being proven today. They have a pictorial and a legendary history. They have a concept of passing through a succession of worlds."

You are suggesting that such concepts do show a capacity for abstract thinking.

Wilkerson: "Yes, but sometimes abstract thought is not the answer to our needs. I think we need to do a little bit of thinking about the process of satisfying needs. But, sure, we delve into the now and the present, and we live for the present and we also live for the past. We know the future and what it holds for us. But we don't put these abstractions in the same kind of concepts that the non-Indian does.

"The Hopi prophecies were made thousands of years ago. We know this takes abstract thinking to do this. We don't deal with the future in the sense that a non-Indian would, but we do consider the future. We do make suppositions about the future, but we don't allow them to become overwhelming in our lives.

"Our manner of abstract thinking takes different forms, so therefore it is not recognized as such by non-Indian people. We do abstract thinking from our own frame of reference, and until you can put yourself into our frame of reference, you will never know the Indian mind.

But consider the logic of this: if we had not had the capacity for abstract thought at the time of the whiteman's arrival, we never would have survived.

"Our thought processes may be of a different order, but they certainly include abstract thinking and abstract reasoning. But we do not think from the materialistic viewpoint. I think this is where we get hung up with the whites. Our Circle of Life concept, for example, is certainly abstract thinking. All things interconnected, all things dependent, all things now coming full circle. People are now preaching this, but it has been with us for thousands of years."

What of the charge that all these concepts were stolen and adapted from the whiteman?

Wilkerson: "I've heard this before also. In so many instances the whiteman puts himself in the position of the returning white god spoken of by many of our legends.

"Let me put this right down to basics. We have symbolism in our beliefs wherein colors take very prominent roles. White, for example, stands for purity, cleanliness, sacredness, and all those good things. The White Painted Lady, who has been interpreted by many non-Indian people to mean, 'Oh, man, here is a white Caucasian lady coming back to save the Indians,' means simply this: The lady in the ceremony wears the color of white because she has been painted with the sacred pollen and therefore appears white. Most Indian people would reject out of hand the notion of a Caucasian god coming to save all Indians.

"Much of our religion was destroyed in the way that many of our tribes were destroyed. It is my own personal viewpoint—but one that I might say is shared by many Indian people—that it was the intent on the part of the Founding Fathers of this country to actually destroy native religion. There is a lot of proof around that a lot of white people fully intended to get rid of those ignorant savages and their paganism.

"I reject paganism as an adjective applied to our native beliefs. I think what we had in the old traditions was a deep appreciation of the psychic forces in the world and a deep appreciation of the Supreme Being. The overwhelming evidence is that the Indian people were very deeply religious."

Mad-wa-sia-win (Joe Northrup), a Chippewa from Cloquet, Minnesota, wrote (in 1931) that his people did most certainly have the concept of the Great Spirit before the arrival of the Christian missionaries:

> In common with other primitive peoples, the Divine Spark or Spirit . . . was in the minds and hearts of these people long before the Christian religion invaded America. They knew of an all pervading force, or as they called this God, the Great Spirit, the one above all spirits; they knew of lesser spirits as well, as the Evil Spirit, whom they feared because this spirit was supposed to hate all Indians and was continually sending evil things upon them.
>
> They worshipped in faith this Great Spirit whom they called 'Ge-Ji-Munido' or Good Spirit and knew him as the author of all good, all life and embodying love and purity in its truest sense.
>
> All life was caused by containing Spirit. Thus the Chippewa believed trees, grass, water, wind, clouds, in fact all things that grew or moved and had life or spirit were subject to the Great Spirit. Therefore, the Chippewa Indian had the utmost respect and reverence for all the forces and beauties of natural life. . . .
>
> The Chippewa, in his native state with inborn piety left him by countless generations of natural sons of the Great Spirit, and his manner of life in nature, therefore, close to nature, imbibed the peace and quiet of the great forests, even in infancy was in closer communion with the mysterious Spirit world. So great was their faith in this unseen world, that all children were compelled at the age of reason, seven years, to fast at least one day, purifying their minds the better to get in tune with this all pervading Force. At the age of twelve came the regular fast or purifying of the mind. . . .
>
> —Courtesy of the Minnesota Historical Society
> Cedar Street and Central Avenue
> St. Paul, Minnesota

In the 1850s, James Lynd, a fur trader acquainted with the ways and language of the Dakota, began the massive task of writing a history of his aboriginal clientele in Minnesota. He had invested several years of effort in this project when Little Crow led the Sioux War; and, according to several accounts, Lynd became the first whiteman killed, on either August 17 or 18, 1862.

The Dakota entered the general store of the fur trader, killed him, and scattered the pages of his manuscript. It remains uncertain whether or not the Indians knew what was written on the pages which they threw about the store; but, the manuscript pages lay scuffed, bloody, and spat upon until a soldier happened to notice what they were and considered the fact that they might have a certain value. James Fletcher Williams compiled a volume from the surviving pages and made a gift of it to the Minnesota Historical Society.

Basing his opinion on many years' observation of the Dakota people, Lynd wrote the following about their belief in the Great Spirit:

> No question has more puzzled—and it may be said, unnecessarily—those who have gone among the Sioux than that of, who the *Wakantanka* or Great Spirit is. Though the name is frequently heard, yet it does not appear to be well understood even by the Sioux themselves: and from the fact that they offer no praise, sacrifices, or feasts to that Divinity, many have gone so far as to imagine that the *name, even was introduced to their acquaintance by the whites!*
>
> Nothing could be more unfounded than this. Not to mention the absurdity of the proposition that so radical an idea as that of one spirit being superior to and more powerful than all others—an idea at the bottom of and pervading all religions, even the most barbarous—should meet with an exception in the Dakota. There are internal proofs of its native origin, both in the testimony of the people, and in the use of the word itself. . . .
>
> We have already seen that the word *Wakantanka* is of frequent occurrence in . . . Sacred Feasts: and that it is used interchangeably with the Algonquin word, *Maneto,* or Great Spirit. This, alone is proof enough; but there are other proofs. In the Medicine Dance, which though very modern as far as the Dakotas are concerned, was introduced among them long years before any Mission reached them; the *Wakantanka* is expressly declared to have been the creator of the world. . . . Further proof is not required.
>
> —Courtesy of the Minnesota Historical Society
> Cedar Street and Central Avenue
> St. Paul, Minnesota

In his aforementioned open letter to the Christian churches, Vine Deloria, Jr., writes:

> Early missionaries . . . told us the story of Adam and Eve. They went on at great length with stories of Jonah and the whale. They regaled us with the accounts of the resurrection, the Exodus, and the Tower of Babel. We recognized these stories as myths by which a people explain how they came to consciousness as a national community. When we tried to explain our myths, the missionaries grew angry, and accused us of believing superstitions.

Superstition is, of course, in the dogma of the beholder. As has long been observed, the god of one spiritual expression has the potential of becoming the devil of another—especially if in the confrontation between religions, one faith has the benefit of being sponsored or cherished by the dominant, or conquering, culture.

George W. Cornell of the Associated Press reports that the Episcopal Church, the United Church of Christ, the American Baptist Convention, and the Lutheran Council in the United States are among those denominations which have set up special Indian departments, directed by Indians, to bolster church sensitivity to American Indian interests.

At a January 1973 meeting of Indians and church leaders held in Estes Park, Colorado, the Reverend Homer Noley, an Indian clergyman who heads United Methodist Indian work, told those assembled that traditional Indian religion is "closer to original Christianity" than most orthodox church people realize. "Our ancestors believed in a spirit world of all things," Reverend Noley commented.

The Reverend Dr. Benjamin Reist, dean of San Francisco Theological Seminary at San Anselmo, California, admitted that Christian theology is "terribly impoverished when it comes to a doctrine of nature," and prognosticated that there must soon come a day when "American Indian theology must be represented in the highest councils of Christian theology in the world."

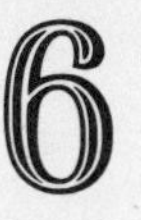

6 Seneca Medicine Woman

> A few hours ride from the railroad station in a wagon, not the easiest, of a road, not the smoothest, meeting narrow escapes as to mudholes and deep ruts, and you will find yourself upon the Cattaraugus Indian Reservation. You might as well be west of the Rocky Mountains for any indications of the Paleface that you see here. Indians on the roads and in the homes, working on the farms and building houses; Indian children with ball-clubs, snow-snakes and arrows; Indian babies upon the backs of their mothers; Indian corn bread boiling in the kettles under the trees; Indians here, there, and everywhere, the straight black hair and shining black eyes that mark the race everywhere meet you here. You hear the curious intonations of their strange language all about you, and yet you are only 30 miles south of Buffalo, and 500 miles from New York City.
>
> —*Our Life Among the Iroquois Indians*
> Mrs. Harriet S. Caswell, 1892

Eighty-one years after Harriet Caswell viewed the scene she described in her book, we were entering a Seneca home on the Cattaraugus Reservation. Although Twylah Nitsch's ancestral home had been constructed after the style of the whiteman in 1858, each succeeding generation had contributed its own new room, new roof, or new siding. Modern appliances, attractive carpeting, and a baby grand piano blended with Native American art and artifacts.

On both her grandfather's as well as her grandmother's side of the family, Twylah is a descendant of the great Seneca chief Red Jacket. Red Jacket was a brilliant orator and a staunch defender of his people's traditions. Twylah has inherited both attributes.

In her study is a cherished portrait of Red Jacket that has been in Twylah's family for years. On the back of the portrait a stylish hand once wrote with quill pen, "Taken from life by Joseph B. Gardner of Nantucket, July 21, 1835."

Shortly after we arrived at the Nitsch home, Twylah invited us to meet a committee that had assembled in a long, low, building nearby to discuss future events of the Seneca Indian Historical Society. The building, we learned as we followed Twylah, had been the original Buffalo Creek longhouse of the Senecas. Twylah's husband Bob had recently remodeled the longhouse into a utilitarian studio for crafts work and classes.

Twylah, together with her mother Maude Hurd and three other Seneca women living on the Cattaraugus Reservation, founded the historical society early in 1970. The brief business meeting was taken up with such matters as how to obtain grants and aids, how best to conduct arts and crafts programs, and, interestingly, how to attract white people to attend functions held on the reservation. Apparently even whites in the area had little knowledge of their Native American neighbors' homelife, and a good many seemed to express a great reluctance, even fear, of entering the reservation.

After the committee had adjourned, Twylah began our interview by asking me a question. "Do you know what 'squaw' means?"

Of course I knew that "squaw" was used in countless motion pictures and popular novels of cowboy-and-Indian fiction as the word denoting the wife of an Indian man. Since there are many diverse American Indian languages and dialects, it is obvious that all tribes did not originally use the word "squaw" to identify the female members of their groups. No doubt the early fur traders had corrupted an eastern tribe's word for woman, and their version of the pronunciation had become standard and universal in its application. However, I had noticed that some American Indian women rankled at the word and seemed to consider its usage as pejorative and Twylah's tone of voice told me that she considered the use of the word to be reprehensible.

"The word probably originally meant a beast of burden," I answered Twylah, taking what I considered to be an educated guess.

Twylah seemed amused, but she frowned and shook her head. "When the fur trappers came on their boats, they had been away from their towns for a long time, and they were looking for women. They couldn't make the Indian men understand what they wanted, so they exposed their genitals and made suggestive movements.

"The Indian men said, 'Oh, *numsquaw,'* giving the word for the male genitals. The traders brightened, thinking they had made themselves understood, and shouted, 'Yeah! Squaw! Squaw! Squaw!'

"So you see, Indian women don't want to be called squaws because they have no right to the word. It has nothing to do with women. I want to get letters off to the dictionary companies, asking them to delete the word. Not to make it an issue, but just to delete squaw from the dictionary. People think it is an Indian word for woman, and it certainly is not."

Satisfied that her point had been made, Twylah turned to a subject very dear to her heart and spirit—her grandfather Moses Shongo, last of the great Seneca medicine doctors:

Twylah: "I would like to tell you that before I was born my grandfather was very worried about who was going to take over the teachings. He had handed his medicine bag to his son. My mother had a child who had died at birth, and it seemed that they were not going to have any more children.

"Eventually, Mother became pregnant. Grandfather and Mother conducted some Indian rituals to make sure that she was in proper condition to carry this child. He would say to her, 'Maybe this child will live and carry on where I have found no one else to do so.'

"I was born, and he said, 'This child will be able to walk on two paths. She has white blood in her, as well as Indian blood; therefore, she will be able to move from the Indian to the white.'

"When I was about two years old, I came down with a very serious case of whooping cough. In those days there were no effective medicines to overcome this. Even today, whooping cough is very hazardous for a young child.

"One night during the course of my illness, I coughed and choked. Mother became frightened, because I was turning blue. She quickly got my grandfather (we all lived together). He used mouth-to-mouth resuscitation, and he brought me around.

"He said to Mother, 'Now she will carry on my work, because my breath is her breath.'

"My mother told me this about a year before she died. Of course, no one had heard about mouth-to-mouth resuscitation at the time, but Grandfather saved my life with it.

"About six months before she died, Mother said, 'I don't know why I am still around. I have taught you everything I know. I don't know what else I can do. I can help much more on the other side.' I said, 'Mother, you must still have something to do.'

"She slept upstairs. She went to bed, and suddenly at the foot of the bed, Grandpa and her brother and grandmother were standing there.

"She said, 'Oh, what are you here for? Did you come for me?'

"They said, 'No, you have to tell Twylah that it is all right. She must do the teaching and the sharing she is thinking about doing. She is not listening to us. She withdraws once it comes to the point of doing it. She has got to do it. We have given this knowledge to her, and we are helping her.'

"Mother came downstairs. She said, 'Twy, I have to tell you what happened.' She told me, and I felt so good. Mother said, 'The time is now.'

"Just prior to Mother's dream, I would go to Rosary Hill College, where I was teaching, with the strongest feeling that I should take Grandpa's stone pestle to class. One day I took it into the house, got some Indian tobacco, ground it, and burned it.

"Mother said, 'You should never have done this.' I said, 'Mom, I had to. Grandpa impressed me to do it.'

"Mother was very upset with me, because she went along to class. She said, 'If you do it right, it will be fine; but you have never done it!" I said I would do it right.

"I conducted a very simple ceremony. I asked Mother to pray. Her prayer was beautiful. On our way home, I said, 'It was all right, wasn't it?' Mother agreed that it was. That class is still talking about that ceremony!

"That experience, together with Mother's dream, was all I needed. From then on, all these things have been coming to me."

Neither your mother nor your father are living today.

"No, my mother passed away two years ago, and my father passed away four years ago. Mother was a very marvelous person. She had a great deal of spiritual depth. My father could have had, but he just didn't get involved in the closeness of the Indian, except to do the craft work and to help with initiations and adoptions. We have had fairs here on this farm all the time. It is a place for people to come. The name was Shongo Farms. Everyone knew the place."

What does shongo mean?

"Shongo is not an Indian name per se. Shongo is a contraction, an abbreviation. It means 'in the spring. . . in the water.'

"Years ago, the Seneca would take the newborn child, place it in spring water to help it draw its first breath. I recall being told that when I was born and I wasn't crying, I was placed in the cold water, just enough to alarm the body."

And this is truly your ancestral home.

"Yes, I was born here. My mother was born here, and I was born on my mother's birthday."

What year did your great-grandfather build the house on this farm?

"Great-grandfather Two Guns started to build it in 1858. He moved in when my grandmother was a baby. When the Seneca came down here, the Deer clan lived on the other side of the road. The Wolf clan lived on this side. Bob was very perturbed because our family didn't adopt him. The Deer clan adopted him so he could be a Deer married to a Wolf. Many Deer married Wolves. You never marry in your clan.

"Jane Pierce was my grandmother. She married Daniel Webster Pierce, who taught in the district school as an educator. She was one of the students. They fell in love. He was a few years older, of course. They had just one daughter, my grandmother. The Indians called her 'that white woman,' because she was a descendant of Mary Jamison, an early white captive of the Senecas. Because the Indians and the white people weren't exactly on good terms, 'white' was a bad word.

"My Grandfather Moses Shongo came from Allegheny, from the Buffalo Creek Reservation. He came up here and married my grandmother. When there is a marriage among Seneca, the women take the husbands to their own homes. Today the lifestyle is somewhat the same. I did the same thing. Bob came to my home.

"We came down here from Buffalo and fixed the place up. Bob didn't know at first, but when the polio epidemic came around, we wanted to get the family out of the city. It was quite a change—no electricity, no running water. Nothing but plain country living. Bob loved it so much, he said he was willing to take a stab at it."

Was there any resentment toward a whiteman living on the reservation?

"My dad was considered white, because he was one-quarter Oneida. His people died when he was very young, and a white family took his sister and him into their home.

"When Dad's Oneida grandmother came to visit, the white family chased her away. They called her a witch. Dad ran away, but they caught him before he could find her. He was only ten years old. When he went into the army, he met my mother's brother, who introduced him to my mother, and they were married.

"When Dad lived down here, people called him a whiteman, too. Even now if someone gets mad at me, they call me a white woman.

"I don't believe there is one family on the reservation that is 100 percent Indian."

How many Indians here on the reservation are following the traditional ways?

"There are very few. They don't know the ways my grandfather taught me. Those teachings are very simple. There are four questions, which also serve as guidelines in self-discipline.

"Ask yourself: 1. Am I happy in what I'm doing? 2. Is what I'm doing adding to the confusion? 3. What am I doing to bring about peace and contentment? 4. How will I be remembered when I am gone?

"If you are with your friends, you ask yourself, am I happy with my friends? If there is a discussion which creates an argument, what did I do to add fuel to the fire? Was I responsible for it? What did I do to bring about peace and contentment? How will I be remembered when I am gone? These questions make a circle. You can keep on going around and around.

"When disciplining a child, ask him if he is happy doing what he is doing. If he is happy doing the naughtiness, he may answer yes. Then explain to him what will happen if he continues. Let him know if he continues, he alone will be responsible. I learned a lot of lessons that way!

"The Indians always believed in one Creator. The energy or the force or the power of the Creator will manifest itself in any possible way. You always pray in thanksgiving for this magnificent force. For this reason, the Indian could embrace the Christian religion. Christ taught brotherly love, and that is what this was. The Indian felt kinship to all creatures. The Indians could accept Christianity in that way.

"When we went to live in the city while I was going to school, I went to every church that we were near. I have been baptized four times, because everyone wanted to save that little Indian girl.

"The Indian never had any religious wars. They recognized one Supreme Force, which dwelt in the Indian and in everything."

You mentioned being baptized four times. Were you or your parents or grandparents ever members of any orthodox, mainstream church?

"Oh, yes, we belonged to the Presbyterian Church. My great-grandfather embraced Christianity, and he was a minister. He preached at the United Mission church over here. There are about fifteen different denominations on this reservation.

"When the different religious sects came to this reservation, the people accepted them. The missionaries were kind people who wanted to do what they could to make the Indian adapt to the new environment in which they so suddenly found themselves.

" In 1800 an Indian fellow by the name of Handsome Lake came up with his Longhouse religion. Of course it is very close to the Bible. He did a service for his people. The other churches offered nothing to the Indian that was compatible with the Indian lifestyle.

"Handsome Lake's religion flourished for about fifteen years while he was teaching. There was a great deal of misunderstanding. It was then that there began to be arguments among Indians about religion. Prior to any other nations coming to this country, the Indians did not have a word for sin.

"There was no punishment from an angry God. The Indian could not understand all the white people coming and telling him that his way of life was wrong, that he couldn't be saved, that his God couldn't do this or that."

Are you a member of an orthodox church today?

"My husband is a Lutheran. When we were married I had been to so many different churches, I thought it better we go to his church. My children were baptized in the Lutheran Church.

"I don't go to any church now, because there is so much politics in all the churches. I have nothing against any of the basic beliefs of the churches, because fundamentally they are the same. I believe everyone is getting to God in his own way.

"I talk to different people who want to search me out, and I hope I can give them just a little something to think about. I hope that I can say something to give them a little more peace of mind and to help them learn a little more about themselves. I have never forced any thought on anyone.

"Whenever I start to speak, I tell people that my presentation is for information only. If I should happen to have a little gift for them to receive that would enrich their lives, fine.

"I surely am not going to argue with anyone. I speak of the Seneca's lifestyle before the whiteman came here. It is no longer in existence, because the lifestyle of the average Seneca today has been blended in with the American culture as much as possible."

When you were a young woman, did you have any difficulty leaving the reservation? Dallas Chief Eagle has said that growing up on a reservation is worse than growing up in a prisoner-of-war camp; because at least in a war camp, one has hope that the war will be over.

"The Pine Ridge Rosebud people have an environmental problem entirely different from ours. The Cattaraugus Indian Reservation and all the other eastern reservations are in urban areas. Our Indians have a much greater chance of using their skills.

"Due to the balance of their existence with nature, Indians are experts in maintaining physical balance. You will find many of the Iroquois who are builders. As the East developed faster than the West, due to a denser population of people, the eastern Indian had a better opportunity to learn trades than did the western Indian.

"Whenever I leave my home to go into the cities, I am tickled to death that I can come home to the reservation.

"The minute I come over the hill, I know there is peace. We lived in the city while I went to school, and every opportunity we had, we came home. This is home."

Even if you had settled in the city, you would still come home.

"You can tell by what Bob said tonight that this is home. His roots are deep in this place. I never prompted him. You can't put words in his mouth. He is devoted to this place. You heard me talking today in our business meeting about the problems we have in getting the whiteman to come to the reservation. There is a certain fear. We don't know why. There doesn't seem to be any problem with the younger generation, but their parents have a fear of coming here.

"An Indian feels safe here. We walk around after dark and leave our doors open. In the city you can't walk around after dark, or you may have something happen to you. There is a different kind of feeling here. There is a spiritual peace that you cannot find in the city.

"We have joined an association of all artists to cover several counties, but the white people are still reluctant to come to the reservation. They will use the excuse 'I thought the craft show was just for Indians.' Yet on the brochures we sent out, it is stated that the show is for everyone. Those whites who do come are delighted that they came. They are like scouts for the wagon train."

Any ideas as to why this situation exists?

"It is because of the cowboy-and-Indian idea. We have people who come on the reservation and expect to find teepees. They will come down and ask, 'Where are the Indians?' It is silly.

"When I go out and lecture, I put on my costume and white people will say to me, 'Do you ever wear any other clothes?'

"In one instance, this woman said, 'I wonder where our speaker is? They said she would be here early.' I had been introduced to her, but she hadn't got my name. Finally the lady next to me said maybe I should be excused to put my costume on. I excused myself and got dressed in costume. As I walked in again, the lady said, 'Oh, there she is. I was sitting across the table from her!' "

I fear that our entire educational process has always portrayed the Indians as a part of America's past. The implication is that Indians don't even exist today.

"It is true, Brad. The Indians of this area have lost much of their heritage. Few can speak the language, but they want to learn it. The historical society is teaching classes in Indian lanugage.

"In the past it has been better not to be identified as an Indian, because it put you in a different class right away. I know; I have been through it. I went to school that way. I was different. Every Indian goes through this.

"Indians like television sets, homes, and their jobs, just like the whites do. The homes on the reservation are beginning to look like any other American homes. The Indian has an inner peace—if he has retained his Indianism. The reason some are ashamed of their Indianism is that there has been so much confusion within their own families."

Your courtship, according to your husband's testimony, had no problems due to your own heritage.

"No, not for him; but his family frowned on it. They were ashamed that their son had left the city and moved to the reservation.

"But before my father-in-law died of cancer, he called me into his room. He said, 'Twy, I have to tell you this. You know, when Bob married you, we were very much disappointed. A father and mother always feel the girl their son marries is never good enough for him. I want to tell you that I can say now that I couldn't have found a better wife for my son.'

"I felt marvelous. All these years he had had this within his heart.

"When we were married, they never asked us to the house. When our picture would be in the paper, my mother-in-law would be asked if that Indian was her daughter-in-law. Now my mother-in-law is helping me in my Indian projects. At Thanksgiving, she stayed four days. It was fun. So you see, this is the blending after all these years. It makes my husband very happy."

What about your children? Do they follow the old ways?

"My daughter Janice is writing Indian clan stories for small folks. The book I have written is for seventh or eighth or possibly ninth grade level. Together, we are going to put it on possibly a fifth grade level. Diane has a little bit, but she is not quite ready. She is still doing her thing. She is a speech therapist. The two boys know all the tricks of the trade and use them in everything that they do. Our older boy is a musician and musician's agent in Florida. He wears his environment [medicine] stone all the time. He wouldn't go without it.

"When he, our son Bob, was in the service—he was in the navy band—I had a vision of him on an ocean liner with sirens sounding all around him. I could see that there was trouble, but that Bob was all right if he stayed right where he was. I kept projecting to him, 'Bob, you're all right. Don't move. Stay where you are!'

"Weeks later I got a letter from him saying, 'Mother, you were so clear. I could see you and I could hear you saying, "Stay where you are!" '

"He had listened to my image, and everything had worked out fine. They had been playing aboard an ocean liner when fire broke out. He just stayed right where he was until things were back under control.

"Bob and I have a thing going. He will telephone me and ask what I want. He knows when I am thinking about him, wanting to talk to him. Both of the boys, Bob and Jim, and I speak freely of these things. Diane will intellectualize, just as her father will. Janice is pretty well into it."

Did you do anything special when they were children to encourage, or to develop, these abilities?

"Yes, we meditated. I want to start working with my grandchildren in the same way. I have had them in my classes, and they say, 'Grandma, when can we do these things again?' "

Do you feel any link between you and your ancestor, Red Jacket?

"Yes, he is with me a lot. I wasn't going to mention this, but you picked it up, I know. My grandmother and grandfather are constantly with me. My mother is, too, if I ask her to come. This is the way the Indian operates: He talks to his people in the Spirit World. I listen to what my people there tell me.

"I feel that my role in this life is to help others help themselves to adapt to their environment and to find themselves so they can obtain peace of mind. If each person could obtain his own peace of mind, he would help the entire world purify itself. Each individual could help change the entire picture."

[Twylah asked me if I had my medicine stone with me. I reached into a pocket, brought forth the small, oblong stone which I carry.]

My daughter Julie gave this to me when she was four years old. She had been outside somewhere, and when she came back into the house, she presented this rather uniquely shaped stone with the announcement that it was to be mine. Since she was at that possessive-ownership age, I assumed something pretty heavy must have told her that this was to be my medicine stone.

Twylah took my stone, held it thoughtfully in an open palm. "Yes, I am sure that this is your stone. But let us find another."

She took two rather large bags from a closet of the longhouse workshop. "Here," she said, dumping their contents on the floor, "choose your stone from among these. Pass your hand over them until one sends out the vibration that it is yours."

I knelt, moved my hands over the stones.

"Open yourself," Twylah admonished. "Open up and let the stones speak to you. When you have selected a stone, I shall read it for you.

"The foundation of the universe is a stone. A stone is a common denominator of the universe. You can find one wherever you go. A stone has form and spirituality. Even the uninitiated have feelings for stones, whether they realize it or not. When this Earth is cleansed, it will be the stone that will be the nucleus and expand or contract. The Indians have a beautiful philosophy that revolves around the stone, and it has almost been lost."

Early missionaries used to bemoan the fact that the Indians worshipped stones.

Twylah smiled, shook her head slowly. Her eyes closed momentarily, as if she were visualizing a memory of a scene that had occurred before her own birth.

"The Indians did not worship the stone. The Indian used the stone to remind him of the oneness of all creatures of the universe and that the same spiritual energy flows through all things.

"Let me recite for you a poem, a song, that came to me about stones. These things come to me, Brad. First a title comes. Then I wait. The song-poem comes in spurts. Through the night, I will dream it. I am not me. I have no image. I am floating around. It is not me, Twylah, writing such things down."

THE BLESSED EVENT

A tiny droplet fell from the cloud,
filled with gifts spiritually endowed.
It descended amidst God's radiance
to seek its earthly residence.

A minute spot of moisture round,
Settled upon the warm soft ground.
Nature's depth of welcoming
Filled it through to envelop him.

The droplet's heart was filled with glee,
For he thought what he would like to be.
Desire struck with a mighty blow
About the gifts that he must know.

Traveling down into the earth,
Telling his wealth within his girth.
To share it with true ecstasy,
Among the creatures he would see.

Soon he heard a thundering roar,
That shook where he stood on the soily floor.
The creatures scattered as fast as they could,
But he didn't move. He stayed where he stood.

The earth heaved and rolled
and spun him around,
The next thing he knew
His spot was unsound.

The earth opened up and down he fell,
Into a steaming, watery well.
He floated around in this dungeon place,
Wondering if this was his resting place.

He looked around and to his surprise,
Droplets like him had the same surmise.
They clung together as they swirled and twirled,
Not knowing where they would next be hurled.

Confusion and tension lurked at their side,
Bringing fear-ridden feelings in a drive to do right.
It came abrupt, their violent encounter,
Walls filled a space and rotted asunder.

All droplets dispersed hither and yon,
Into unknown cracks and fissures beyond.
A droplet fell through a darkened abyss,
Hitting out jutted rocks, he just couldn't miss.

He tried to touch the slippery wall,
There was nothing to grasp to break his fall.

Terrified thoughts raced through his mind.
Was he to live in a place of this kind?
Tumbling, falling, not knowing where,
Or did the Creator not really care?

When suddenly from way down below,
A shimmering ray began to glow.
Its radiance burst to a brilliant light
In a rainbow of colors; what a glorious sight.

He splashed upon a rocky place,
Where God caressed him in a spiritual embrace.
His terrified thoughts no longer could live,
For God had filled him with his love to give.

He nestled into a shiny stone,
Immediately, he knew this was his home.
Pressed deeply into the soul of Mother Earth,
He would be nurtured to await his rebirth.

God's radiance of love was felt and seen,
For the rocks were sharing his essence supreme.
If only we could glow and shine like them.
"You can," saith God, at a birth of a gem.

From the Teachings of Twylah

"It is time to commune with nature." These were the words that opened the way for Seneca Indian instruction. The teacher was Moses Shongo, the last of the Seneca medicine doctors. I can see him now sitting on the porch of our home on the Cattaraugus Indian Reservation. I sat on one of the stone slabs which served as steps leading to the entrance of our home.

The white, rambling farmhouse was my birthplace. It was built by my great-grandfather in 1858 after the Senecas lost their beloved Buffalo Reservation. The house stood like the hub of a wheel with the majestic sugar maples nodding in the gentle breeze.

Our home was designed so that the forces of nature streamed through from the east to west, from the back door to the front, as the Sun traveled the sky path. My grandfather's chair occupied the north corner of the porch. It wrapped around his bulky form as he snuggled down upon its squeaky springs. When he was deep in thought, his fingers tapped rhythmically on the armrest.

I watched him in profound wonderment and followed him in action every day. My eyes were drawn to the tanned fedora hat that had acquired a personality all its own. A crop of jet-black hair, shiny as a raven, peaked beneath the brim of his hat. His sparkling eyes were pools of wisdom, transmitting his innate love. While his face beamed with a smile, it radiated spiritual brotherhood. He could be likened to a big tree, the greatest compliment of our ancestors. He stood proud and erect, looking deep into the essence of Mother Earth, always affirming thanksgiving for her gifts.

At the close of each day, facing the west, he watched the Sun, the center of our universe, slowly descend beyond the trees. "Prepare yourself for the lessons of the Great Spirit," Grandfather would say. My eyes beheld the burning aura, silently sinking to the rim of the sky. A glorious sensation prepared me for the sanctity of the Sky Dome, the place of spiritual tranquility. An ebon essence brushed across my face, as I was borne aloft.

The Golden Dome, abounding in iridescent splendor, filled my senses with vitalizing awareness. Then, a whisper, steeped in solemnity, echoed within me. It was the voice of the Great Spirit.

I had prepared myself well, as I had been taught, and I was ready for whatever Grandfather was inspired to tell me. I can hear his strong voice now, speaking to me of the ways of our people.

In his learned way, as his ancestors taught, he woud say, "Long before there was time, place, or even human beings, there was a Great Spirit." I cannot recall a time when this statement did not preface the lessons I was to hear. It rings in my mind to this day, filling me with the peace and reverence that only spiritual feeling can express.

Many long years ago, our ancestors trod paths along the animal trails that had been made before them. These passageways carved the shortest and safest distances between neighboring villages and distant nations, where Indians traveled to exchange cultural views, customs, and traditions.

The wisdom of life is learned from the greatest teacher, Mother Earth.

Countless examples of nature's perfection, splendor, and harmony are manifested all around the early Indians. A central wisdom, known by all medicine doctors as a secret of the ages, asserts that self-understanding is a *desire;* that self-discipline is a *key;* self-control, a *way;* self-realization, the *goal.* The word that encompassed the secret is *communication.* There is a belief that everyone in every nation still acts as a guardian over this secret.

I recall that one of the greatest lessons my grandfather ever taught me was a discussion of the principles that were followed to promote personal happiness among the early Seneca.

"How well do you communicate?" was the question he asked, in his soft, even-modulated voice. "Communicating is understanding. Understanding leads toward peace of mind. Peace of mind leads toward happiness. Happiness is communicating."

These four statements constitute the symbolism of the circle, which embodies spiritual harmony. If problems should arise in your life, the blame can be placed on a lack of communication. We communicate in various ways with every breath we take. Personal happiness should stem from principles developed through routines of daily living regarding the ways we communicate.

A breakdown in personal communication, in many cases, will cause four reactions: anger; withdrawal from the person or the situation that influenced the breakdown; flight, running away from the person or situation identified with the breakdown; the creation of excuses for not facing the situation in order to solve it.

These reactions fall under the heading of immaturity. Immaturity is the basic reason for failure in life, school, work, family, or marriage. No one wants to admit to being immature, yet our reactions may reflect such a condition in spite of ourselves.

The following are two thoughts of wisdom: We cannot reap happiness while wallowing in the mire of immaturity, because immaturity fosters emotional chaos, self-degradation, and depravity. Immaturity permits thoughts of guilt to be nurtured with seeds of peace and love.

The question is, what can we do about immaturity? The first step is to recognize that a problem exists. If a breach occurs in your lifestyle, there is a problem. A breach is any rupture that causes a situation, a separation, insecurity, or disharmony.

Carefully study the four reactions. Can you identify them as belonging to you? If you can, the first step has been faced. At this point, you have recognized that an inner force is available to help you reinforce your desire for making an honest self-analysis. You have tapped into your creative mind, your place of highest gift. Everyone possesses this gift and the ability to use it—that is, if the individual has the desire to solve the problem.

The longer a problem is allowed to exist, the harder it is to return to peace of mind. When a problem exists, you tend to bring others to the dilemma. It takes self-discipline to face and to accept the blame for causing a problem to exist. Our thoughts and actions account for our living in a state of conflict. Such a state results in mental restlessness and often illness. Our thoughts can drain our physical energy.

Set the controls with self-discipline and by sharing the best of yourself with others, travel the road with peace of mind. In order to measure your ability to communicate, self-awareness must be sharpened. You do this by tapping into your highest intellectual or creative mind. Then, you understand how to enjoy peace of mind, general good health, and gain self-satisfaction—not only within yourself, but within others who are in your environment.

The second step is to adapt yourself to faith. We are not born in faith. It is a characteristic that must be developed. Faith needs to dwell within as a part of our nature before we can sincerely enjoy sharing it with others. It is the sharing that brings the most happiness and the feeling of well-being.

Parents play a vital role in developing faith patterns in their children. Because some parents do not inject faithful characteristics in their daily lives, they tend to tear down, rather than build, faith in their children. We learn through example. For this reason, take time to evaluate the home environment that helps establish your way of life.

You may recognize extending a bad state of affairs into your life from the unthinking examples affecting your personal development. To accept this unthinking shows a lack of maturity.

Successful communication depends on self-understanding and a reasonable amount of faith. Only when personal faith patterns have been developed can we find what pressures and tensions have the ability to devour a secure image.

When a dimension of faith is lost, we withdraw into a shell of self-pity, caring for nothing, not even for ourselves. We live out our lives in personal thought patterns that serve as habits and behavior traits. When these thought patterns fall into undesirable habits, they rob us of peace of mind and health; and, they often bring on creative confusion that affects those who happen to be under our influence. Measuring our abilities to communicate self-awareness must be sharpened. I emphasize this because it is so important.

Free yourself from negative influence. Negative thoughts are the old habits that gnaw at the roots of the soul. When these negative habits flare up, counteract them by flooding your mind with a powerful thought, one that disciplines your personality. It is incredible how this technique has the power to reinforce the positive action. The more this technique is practiced, the easier the negative thought is erased. A surge of new confidence and strength will stream through your body, as this achievement takes hold.

Self-realization is the goal; put this affirmation at the tip of your tongue. Nurture these words of wisdom and make them part of your lifestyle. Such an affirmation is the umbilical cord of creativity. You are born with the ability to attain self-realization. There is no reason for your failure in lifestyle, because, by this lesson, you have been enlightened to see that wisdom is yours to use.

This brought to an end one of the greatest lessons my grandfather ever taught. If it had not been for this lesson and the wisdom of my people, I would have been crushed beneath the vibrations of immature people I have met and smothered with my own self-indulgent rituals of immaturity. I am sharing this wisdom and spiritual insight with you, feeling secure that the infinite Great Spirit guides you and tells you what to do.

Before any human beings, there was the Great Spirit.

After preparing the Sun and Moon and Water and setting them into place, the Great Spirit made patterns for all things which were to be born and arranged for all happenings which were to occur. Then the Great Spirit prepared Nature Land where all things were to mingle in harmony. Next the Great Spirit caused creatures to be evolved, from plants to creatures that swam, crawled, walked, and flew. As they evolved, gifts were bestowed upon them with abilities to learn lessons from one another.

All things are sent and belong to the Great Spirit. For this reason, the Spirit is in everything that breathes, senses, hears, tastes, smells, and sees. The Spirit is in all emotions; it is present at birth and at death. The inhabitants of Nature Land are aware of the Great Spirit through the whisperings that speak through the mind.

It is time to commune with Nature; Her knowledge of life we drink.
She lays her wealth before us, and hopes that we'll learn to think.
We're filled with events for learning;
When comforts brought ease, it dimmed our yearning.

In the very beginning, the Seneca were drawn close to nature. Legends related the wonders of nature and its effect on all creatures and plants. It was not long before the ancestors of the Senecas sensed a powerful force revealed all around them. Some were able to feel the force; others were able to see it. They called the force *Swen-i-o,* the Great Mystery.

The lessons nature taught set a pattern for Senecas to follow. They soon learned that each Indian must find a way to fit into this pattern in order to experience a sense of happiness. By the process of trial and error, a series of techniques evolved that helped the people develop a thorough and more meaningful use of their minds.

In the atmosphere of the forest, they recognized the presence of the Great Mystery. Its force penetrated into every soul, making every soul a part of it. This was where nature influenced the life of the early Senecas. This rhythm blended all creatures into complete harmony, instilling the habitual silence of the Seneca as a characteristic.

When alone with his thoughts, he listened and heard the Silence.
He listened and saw the Silence.
He listened and tasted the Silence.
He closed his eyes and felt the Silence deep within.
The woodlands became his chapel; his body, the altar.

In the Silence, he began to communicate with his Creator, and he received peace.

In solitude, he felt his thoughts being guided to a higher intellectual level. The feeling of belonging to nature brought him back, time and time again, to be enchanted by the Great Mystery.

It was only natural that the early people sought these quiet moments, for it was their first realization of spiritual love. Nature was Mother Earth, the caretaker of all creatures and plants. They needed to share her gifts with others in faith, work, love, and pleasure.

Learning the unspoken language of the inhabitants who live in the forest helped the Seneca to understand the necessity for having a purpose in life—to live in harmony with self and with nature. The Senecas accepted the kinship of all creatures and plants of nature. The Senecas believed all creatures and plants were equal in the eyes of nature, each performing its specific talents according to its abilities.

Whenever the Seneca fell out of balance with nature, they caused conditions of discord. Discord caused the illnesses, frustrations, and disasters that visited them. When the Seneca developed spiritual equality and a life of spiritual balance, they became a mature people of wisdom.

The Seneca taught their children the importance of identifying themselves with all creatures and plants of nature. This was the first step in helping the children to see the problems that all creatures and plants must overcome in order to stay in harmony with nature. They learned the difference between the creatures, but they felt the same spirit flowing throughout all of them.

Feeling to the Seneca can be described as his faith. The depth of his feeling was measured by the depth of his faith. Learning how to identify this depth depended upon the ability to recognize the different levels of feeling through self-knowledge.

The early Seneca recognized that there was a spiritual feeling and a material feeling. Spiritual feeling can be unlimited, whereas material feeling has its limitations. In the spiritual level dwelt all desires. Material feelings were a result of material experiences relying upon the senses—seeing, hearing, smelling, and tasting.

One of the methods used to understand spiritual feelings as compared with material feelings is as follows:

Close your eyes and look straight ahead. Look out behind the eyelids. These are the spiritual eyes. What you see depends upon your personal experiences. Open your eyes, and these are the material eyes. Many times they fool you.

The second step is to listen for your heartbeat. Become aware of the feelings you experience while listening to your heartbeat. This is going within. This is when you realize that maybe your heartbeat is becoming a little less pronounced. And then you establish a balance within yourself. This balance is the point of relaxation where you feel comfortable. Everyone can find this.

Open your eyes, and make a self-evaluation of what you've accomplished.

Faith was the first stepping stone that led toward love, work, and eventually pleasure. Faith gave a strong feeling of belonging to something, or someone. In the beginning, the something was Mother Earth. All Indians had faith in Mother Earth.

A small child nestled in its mother's protective arms feels the first level of faith. As faith grows, the depth of feeling becomes evident. The physical contact of mother and child causes faith to flow between them, as feeling. Therefore, feeling needs to be present to express the first stages of faith.

The habit of being faithful was considered on a spiritual level. All forms of creativity were believed to be gifts of the Creator. If these habits had their roots in the spiritual level, creativeness and actions were more easily controlled—and were better understood.

Because faith had become established and feeling was present, adding the ingredient of warmth led to love. Where there was no feeling, there was no fath; so, faith and feeling appeared to go hand in hand. To the Seneca Indian, extending the open hand became a symbol of faith. The degree of faith began to manifest itself by different degrees of warmth.

To the early Seneca, love was a feeling that had grown from the seed of faith. The degree of love was measured by the feeling of warmth. The Sun was revered by the Indians because of its love for the nature people. It shared its warmth with them. Through self-discipline the Indian had to control the amount of love he accepted from nature, as well as that which he was willing and able to share with others. You have to know how much warmth you can accept—or you will be burned to a crisp.

Love, faith, and work cannot be measured without feeling. The level of hearing, seeing, smelling, and tasting cannot be measured without a degree of feeling. Faith, nourished with deep feeling, developed the warmth of love. Continued faithful actions on the part of an individual toward others created good feelings. Its warmth could be felt when people assembled.

The feeling of warmth appeared more intense between a mother and her child. It was always present where families gathered. Faith and warm love lived together. Where one was, you could always find the other. The Sun, therefore, was a symbol of love to the early Seneca.

The circle, the shape of the Sun, took on an added significance; it was symbolic of perfection and equality. The Sun's color was the most revered because of its beauty and magnificence. The Indians found themselves smiling whenever the Sun shone upon them. They believed that the Sun smiled at them all the time.

Smiling at someone and placing one's hand in another's signified the presence of love. To smile at someone was to convey a spiritual message of good will. Words were not always necessary where faith and love were present. The feelings that accompany love speak for themselves.

The Senecas held a fixed purpose in life, and that was to learn about the Great Mystery. To them, the Great Spirit was the Great Mystery.

The Great Spirit—the Divine Supreme, Maker of All Things, Now and Forever.

The Great Spirit—the Eternal Mind, whose thoughts flow everlastingly.

The Great Spirit—the Master Designer, the Arranger of Patterns of All and Everything.

The Great Spirit—the Celestial Law, the Perpetuator of Perfection.

The Great Spirit—the Ethereal Voice, the Composer of the Harmony in Nature.

The Great Spirit—the Great Mystery, God.

Going into the Silence meant communing with nature in spirit, mind, and body. Nature's atmosphere radiated the spirituality of the Supreme Power and provided the path that led the early Seneca into the Great Silence.

The legend of the First Messenger of Swen-i-o, the Great Mystery, tells of the encounter with the spiritual essence that was responsible for the practice of going into the Silence.

Four very old people, two men and two women who were endowed with great wisdom gleaned throughout their advancing years, sat in the woodlands on the warm earth near a brooklet that crept beneath a canopy of leaves and branches. They had come to reminisce of their kindred experiences when suddenly the heavens opened:

A Glorious Beam of Light
In All Its Brilliant Splendor
Gently Drifted Over Them
Seeding Peace and Solemnity
On Everything It Touched.

They watched in wonderment, spellbound by the Light's sublime magnificence. It filtered through their bodies, cleansing them of all infirmities.

Presently, they were borne aloft to a place of divine ecstasy, where the "Secret of the Ages" was revealed to them, telling of things to be. They saw the first messenger of the Supreme Power: the spiritual hand with outstretched fingers and thumb. The message was *Ens-wy-stawg,* meaning, "It comes through." This was the first spiritual experience of "going into Silence."

The symbolism of the hand signifies that as the thumb assists the four fingers in life, unity, equality, and eternity, so does the Supreme Power or Great Spirit assist all things in nature.

From that time on, the four people of wisdom spent their remaining days communing with nature in reverence and solitude. Their spiritual insight increased as others joined them to listen to their words of wisdom and spiritual counseling.

From this revelation the entire custom of sitting in council evolved. It became evident that the messengers of the Great Spirit wore many faces. They could be manifestations of nature, creatures, or earthly forces.

The Secret of the Ages revolved around attitudes and thoughts that instilled a sense of brotherhood with all creation. Its practice was carried on as a personal attribute in solitude with one's own thoughts in direct communication with the Creator. It mattered not when or where it was held, since the body was the chapel that housed the spiritual light.

The following procedure was found to be helpful in entering the Silence:

The Indian discovered that wherever he went he could find a stone. After selecting one of his choice, the stone was placed in the palm of the left hand with the right hand clasped on top. Holding the stone in this fashion created a union of forces within the hand. When this pulsating was felt, the Indian believed he had raised himself into the vibrational current of a higher spiritual level. The stone acted as a reminder that everything was of the same source—the spiritual brotherhood of all and everything.

The following mental procedure was also useful in entering the Silence. It helped the Indian locate a place in his mind where peace and contentment lived.

You are walking into the woods. Your feet are plotting a path on the soft, spongy ground. The path is narrow and winds around trees and bushes so that, at times, you need to duck under the low-hanging branches.

Through the clearing ahead lies a shimmering lake. The Sun spreads a rainbow of colors across the rippling surface.

Upon reaching the water's edge, you stand quietly and listen to the lapping surf as it pushes the pebbles back and forth on the clean, warm sand. To the left is a log inviting you to sit upon its blanket of moss. You accept the invitation and settle down upon the cushioned softness, feeling it press against your body. A breeze carrying the woodland aromas brushes your hair and caresses your face. The trees are singing the songs of nature in harmony.

The Silence majestically weaves its magic spell, as it gathers all nature within its fold. At last, the serenity of spiritual Silence flows into your every fiber, drenching it with divine purity.

You listen and hear the Silence.
You listen and see the Silence.
You listen and smell the Silence.
You listen and taste the Silence.
You listen and feel the embrace of the Silence.

Peering through the spiritual eyes, you find the real you dwelling therein. While drifting along with the ebbing tide of spirituality, you and nature become one, together plucking these tender moments of intimate reunion with the Supreme Power, the Great Spirit.

The Great Spirit, Divine Supreme
Maker of all and everything.
The Great Spirit, the Eternal Mind
Whose thoughts flow everlastingly.
The Great Spirit, the Master Designer
Arranger of patterns of all and everything.

Faith in oneself makes work an enjoyment; adventures in knowledge lead toward attunement.

Nature's caretaker is Mother Earth
Her gifts of provision begin at each birth.
We learn from our forebears the secret of use
Obeying these guidelines prevents self-abuse.

Why is the number four sacred to the American Indian?

Twylah: "Remember when the four ancient ones ascended in the Light to the Great Mystery and saw the extended hand?

"They learned that the symbolism of four was present in this extended hand; it meant life, unity, equality, and eternity. It also meant seeing, smelling, tasting, and hearing. These four senses could not function without feeling. Feeling includes touch and all emotion. When the hand is clasped, it is the symbol of unity. Unity is the spiritual law that binds the entire universe.

"They descended with a feeling of being completely healed of all the thoughts they had that were not right. From this experience they saw how the Pathway of Peace should be followed and how the great lessons should be learned. They learned at this time that self-knowledge was the key; self-understanding was the desire; self-control was the way; and, self-realization was the goal.

"They discovered that everything goes in a circle, and that communication is the key to the pathway of learning. They learned communication means understanding; understanding means peace of mind; peace of mind leads toward happiness; therefore, happiness is communicating. A circle again!

"And consider these symbolic representations of the number four:

The first four Creations were Sun, Moon, Water, and Earth.
The four laws of Creation are life, unity, equality, and eternity.
The four seasons are spring, summer, fall, and winter.
The four directions are east, north, west, and south.
The four races of Creation are white, red, yellow, and black.
The four senses of feeling are seeing, hearing, tasting, and smelling.
The four guidelines toward self-development are the following:
Am I happy doing what I am doing?
What am I doing to add to the confusion?
What am I doing to bring about peace and contentment?
How will I be remembered when I am gone—in absence and in death?

The four requirements of good health are food, sleep, cleanliness, and good thoughts.

The four divisions of nature are spirit, mind, body, and life.

The four divisions of goals are faith, love, work, and pleasure.

The four ages of development are the learning age, the age of adoption, the age of improvement, and the age of wisdom.

The four expressions of sharing are making others feel you care; an expression of interest (Everything in creation has something to offer; listen and learn); an expression of friendship (promotes spiritual growth); an expression of belonging (sharing of goals toward a higher spiritual growth).

"My grandfather, Moses Shongo, spent much time breaking things down into fours. He taught me to do things in fours, and all my life I have done this. When I iron clothes, I iron in fours. I iron four things and put them away. Then four more. When I clean, I clean in fours. If I don't do things this way, I don't feel good. If I don't satisfy myself in doing something, I don't bother doing it. It is amazing how it works.

"Unity is the great spiritual law, and we can break that down into four parts, as well:

1. Unity is going into the Silence in spirit, mind, and body.
2. It is a union through which all spirituality flows.
3. It is a goal toward communicating with all things in nature.
4. It is recognized by the intellect through the senses, through the emotions, and through impressions.

"Unity is the law of nature. I have known this since I can remember. Everything has its place, and everything works in unison. If you get into trouble, it is because you have created some static in this unified picture. You have only yourself to deal with. You only have control over yourself; therefore, you have to begin there. Equality to the Indian meant that everything in this universe had a place."

7
A Class Session in a Seneca Longhouse

There were perhaps twenty of us, brothers and sisters. We were gathered in the original Seneca longhouse of the old Buffalo Creek Reservation. Our teacher was Twylah Nitsch, a woman wise in the traditional ways of her people, a woman totally imbued with Seneca wisdom.

Earlier that day Twylah had shared with us her private medicine place. We had walked with her in the autumn-like warmth of an early December day and followed her through the woods until we had come to a place on the side of a hill where a spring bubbled and flowed toward a grassy meadow. This was Twylah's favorite place for going into the Silence. This was also where she replenished her spirit and received insights from the Great Mystery.

Now she stood before us as an instructor, gently authoritative and smilingly firm. There was no question who was in charge.

Twylah pushed the "play" button of a cassette recorder and released the haunting music that had come to her in a vision from the Great Mystery. A friend had played the piece on an organ after transcribing it from Twylah's humming and singing; now the captured tones guided us through the first phase of our class session in a Seneca longhouse.

"Walk to the music," Twylah told us. "Drop off at a chair that is in a place that feels comfortable to you. In order to do what we're going to do tonight, we want everyone to feel very, very comfortable."

As we walked about the longhouse, one did not need to be a psychometrist (one who feels and interprets psychically the history of an inanimate object) to sense the vibrations of the invisible tribesmen of the great Iroquois Nation who moved their feet in cadence with our own. Grandfathers and grandmothers who had long since—in Earth time—passed to the Spirit World returned to their old longhouse that night to join us in a sharing of Seneca wisdom.

After everyone had selected a place, Twylah began:

"I explained to you last week about the seven stones, and that the seven stones are radiating color. As we step on these stones, we will be able to feel the color, and perhaps see it. We will work on this with four senses: the sense of hearing, the sense of tasting, the sense of smelling, and the sense of seeing.

"In some of the classes that I have been conducting, we have experimented to find which way is the most successful for each of us. So we're going to do this tonight, to reaffirm which procedure will be the best for each individual. Some of you, I know, have had experience in seeing. I know some of you know exactly what you are going to do. But there are others who have not experienced those things, especially the young people here. And I'm delighted to have them here, because the young people have not developed so many inhibitions as the oldsters have. For this reason, they will perhaps remember this experience tonight all their lives. So we will start.

"Feel the spiritual light flow into your feet. You can feel your body begin to fill up as a vessel, as spiritual light flows up through your legs. Now I'm not going to tell you how fast it flows, because this is what you will be doing. I'm simply telling you it flows up your body, up to the top of your head.

"From this point your entire body is completely filled with the spiritual light, and it begins to radiate out as far as you want it to, which is usually the distance of your arms outstretched at the top of your head, and you describe a circle within this area. But please do not limit it. This is a rekindling of the spiritual light, and it makes you aware of the spiritual essence that is constantly present within your physical body.

"After you have done this, think of the sounds that you hear. Then think of the taste that you are aware of. So it's what you hear first, then what you taste, and after that, what you smell. Last, what you can see.

"And when you look, keep your eyes closed and look out the back of your eyelids. These are your spiritual eyes, and what you see is unlimited.

"After you have gone through these four stages, decide which is the best procedure for you to become completely relaxed and to feel yourself begin to walk on the Pathway of Peace.

"We will do this in silence for a while, and then I will explain the Pathway of Peace.

"This is what you need to do in order to feel the creative essence flowing within your physical body. We will now stand at the threshold of the Pathway of Peace.

"There are seven stones. Each stone will have a certain radiance. As you step upon the first stone, which has seven sides, you will stand there, and you will request the assistance of a messenger of the Creator—or, if you like, a spiritual hand. You never walk alone. The spiritual hand is always there to assist you.

"You step upon the first stone, and a color will come to you. You remain there until you feel you are ready to step onto the second stone. Each time you step on a stone, another color will manifest itself.

"As you step from one stone to another, you will eventually reach the seventh stone. This stone will be radiating a color similar to violet. You are at the doorway of entering the Silence.

"You may be able to walk the path very fast; but let the impressions come through just exactly the way you feel. When you reach the seventh step, you have opened yourself up to the flow of the Infinite Spirit, and you are then ready for any revelation or gift to be presented to you.

"Each one will do as he feels in going into the Silence.

"We will now sit in complete silence. Try to proceed the best way you can.

"When you have reached the point you wish, come back the way that suits you best. When you again reach the bottom, or the first stone, and you step back into the material world, say a prayer of thanksgiving for this wonderful experience.

"In ancient times, when students wanted to follow a path, they would go to a teacher. He or she would suggest to them the same as I have to you. I would have you find your own way to walk on the stones. Each one of you has a way.

"Don't let color disturb you. This may be all you get. It is good.

"There isn't anything that is bad.

"I can't emphasize this enough. Every experience is emotional. When you feel it emotionally, you have been taught a lesson.

"In spite of the fact that you may say you are not doing it well, you are learning."

Each person went into the Silence, employing Twylah's meditative technique of visualizing the seven stepping stones to the Spirit. After several minutes had passed, Twylah recalled us to the reality we shared on the earth plane. She asked each person to tell what feeling had predominated—hearing, smelling, tasting, seeing—and to describe the colors in which the stones had appeared. Upon the completion of each recitation, Twylah would interpret the meaning of the colors and the things seen, heard, smelled, or tasted by the student.

"Now we are going to do something entirely different. I am going to play the music; as you listen, let yourself go. I am not going to talk. There will be another experience. I hope this will help you understand yourself better."

Twylah punched the cassette and the strains of her song once more filled the longhouse with most remarkable vibrations. After playing the tape through and permitting us to sit for several minutes in silence, Twylah called for us to present our responses and experiences. Again she offered interpretations of the symbols we received.

"One time in class, I used these words to help suggest feeling: as you walk on the soft ground, you can feel the leaves beneath you. You have to duck as you walk beneath the low branches. You look ahead and you see a lake, and you see the Sun with different reflections on the lake. You sit on a log. Feel the soft moss pressing against your body. Smell the aroma that is around you. You get your various senses going, and then you feel yourself floating up and up. You see the real you.

"At the end I asked the people to open their eyes. They all sat there. I waited a little bit and asked them again. No one responded. I waited a little longer, and I wondered what was going on. Finally a girl in the corner said, 'Why don't you shut up! I have never had such a wonderful experience.'

"Another time when I used this music, a young man in the class began to cry. I asked him what the problem was. He said it made him feel sad. I said, 'It certainly isn't sad music to my ears.' He said, 'It is life. It is life in my ears.'

"These are different experiences of the music for different people. There are different moods of the music throughout. I think this music was given to me through my grandfather. He was a wonderful musician. He taught music at Albuquerque.

"In order to make going into the Silence easier to accomplish, I suggest the "four p's": purpose, preparation, procedure, and progression.

"The purpose of going into the Silence is to establish a personal routine that will become a regular experience for spiritual enrichment in your lifestyle. Everyone is searching for personal enrichment. How one goes about it depends on the individual.

"The preparation is so important for this solitary meditation that it should be done as carefully as we prepare our food. Spiritual nourishment is the result, and it is really not only the lifeline, but a guideline for our very existence. It seems the more we become aware of our potential, the more we have the opportunity to enjoy peace. Of course, the best procedure is whichever way you can determine that best helps you to obtain this feeling of ecstasy.

"To the Seneca going into the Silence means a cleansing of feelings which are brought in by his environment.

"During this time the physical body goes through a state of being cleansed and renewed. This is the important thing. Not only to be cleansed, but to be renewed.

"We must resist those thoughts and actions which limit spiritual cleansing. We constantly are resisting things without even thinking.

"The disciplined person entertains feelings that contribute toward his happiness. Feelings are believed responsible for actions in Seneca life and are considered the real motivations behind one's desire. It is necessary to maintain a physical balance between nature and oneself in order to receive spiritual cleansing in spirit, mind, and body. Balance between self and nature is an individual feeling where one feels satisfaction. This is where you have to find that you are satisfied.

"This seeking of balance is constantly affecting you, and your emotions are going up and down. As a result, the physical body is trying to adjust to these emotions. After a while your physical body is drained and you don't know why.

"That brings up something else—streams of energy. The moment you recognize that your energy has been drained, you have raised yourself to a high spiritual level where you can do something about it. If you have never been introduced to the fact that people and things can drain your energy, you can go along and wonder what is the matter with you. You are tired; you become irritable; then your body suffers, because its functioning level has been lowered. Now what do you do? The moment you see or feel that your energy has been drained, look around and see what did it. If there are people around, look about and see who did it. Nine times out of ten, the person who drained your energy is uplifted.

"You will find in an office situation that there are usually two people who drain everyone else's energy. This is my observation. When the two people come to work, they are tired. After they have been on the job awhile, they begin to perk up. They are gnawing away, sniping; but, they are becoming energized.

"You can do something about it. The moment you feel the draining of energy, counteract it by sending a very powerful good thought to them. If they turn around and call you a dirty name, you turn around and send them a good thought.

"I have developed this technique, and it really works: When someone is agitated and they are uptight and things are really bad, *I mentally put them into a drain tile!* The drain tile completely covers them, and I can't see their heads. It is open at the top and at the bottom. The drain tile, in my mind, opens them up to the spiritual essence and permits it to enter the physical body. There is a big sign on the drain tile so everyone can understand it: "With God's Help." It works.

"One of my students works at a bank. She said Friday had been a very difficult day; she felt that she couldn't take another customer. She suddenly realized that she had been drained of much energy—not only from people, but from the job. She put the 'closed' sign on the teller's window, then walked over to the outside window and looked up into the sky. She felt energy come down.

" 'I had my eyes open and all of a sudden I was radiant,' she told me. 'I could feel myself tingling. My head went up and my back went straight. I walked back to my desk. I sat there, because it was such a magnificent feeling.'

"She told this at a meeting, and someone asked her if she became tired again after a while. She said that whenever she felt herself beginning to be drained and whenever she could feel herself going, she experienced a sudden surge of energy. Her head went back, and her back went straight, and she was all right again. She did this several times throughout the day. She said, 'It was I, not the Great Spirit, that was draining my energy.'

"I emphasize, the moment you realize that you have been drained of energy, do something about it, because that is when you can do something about it.

"Plastic bags work, too. You can put yourself into a bag so nothing can get at you. You can visualize anything. I used to say in the hospital, 'If things get really rough, put yourself in a plastic bag.' And nurses would come to me and say, 'It really works!'

"My grandfather's technique was to look at someone and ask him to sparkle his eyes. This is absolutely the most marvelous way to make your audience and your friends feel great. Sometimes at the start of a lecture, I will say, 'Look at your neighbor and make him sparkle!' Then I will say, 'Your eyes are the mirror of your soul. When you sparkle your eyes, whether you think you are beautiful or not, you are.'

"My grandfather would get me agitated and then tell me to sparkle my eyes. I would get so disgusted! I would turn away, but I would always end up looking at him and smiling.

"When your situation is draining you of energy, ask yourself these four questions:

Am I happy with the situation? (Obviously, you are not.)

What am I doing to keep the situation alive? Maybe you are not doing a thing, but because you are doing nothing, you are keeping it alive.

What can I do to change the situation?

If I change the situation, how will it affect the other people around me? Does the situation bother other people as it bothers me?

"Once the boss went away and left an unfinished job on a desk. He was gone a month. We couldn't use the desk because it was cluttered. Everyone had to walk around it because we were afraid of his wrath. If this was such an important project, it would have been handled before he left. No one touched it. It created a bad situation. When the boss returned, he stormed all over the place because the work hadn't been completed. Yet before he left he had told everyone not to touch the work; he would take care of it when he returned.

"This was a classic example of a situation with which no one was happy. So we added to the confusion. No one did anything constructive to bring about peace and contentment. We certainly had fierce thoughts about the boss at the time this was creating confusion.

"Every office has something in it that creates confusion. It might just be where the telephone, wastebasket, or desk is situated. It might be something that needs just a little adjustment.

"The main thing is that you use your creative self to bring about peace and contentment. It keeps your energy level high. Use the best you have. After you have maintained such a habit, it will work better for you. Never, never try to come up with three or four things to do at once. Take one thing at a time. So, that's about draining energy.

"What we have done tonight is to accept the healing forces of the universal spiritual energy that flows through everything and is everywhere. We will close our eyes, and join hands in a circle. Left hand up, right hand down.

"The first thing we do now is to think of someone who probably wouldn't necessarily be what we call a friend. Someone whom we wouldn't even care to have as a friend. Now we send thoughts of healing to him. After we have done this, we think of a loved one to whom we will send the healing forces.

"We are going to close."

> Many moons have traveled the Sky Dome.
> Many moons have followed its course.
> Many lives have evolved before us, guided by your spiritual force.
> The Secret of the Ages is to live in balance, to master all of our inborn talents.
> At the close of each day, in thoughts of thanksgiving we reverently say:
> Thank you, Great Spirit, for the radiant light that heals each body throughout this night.

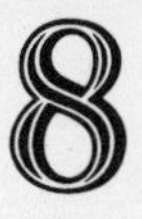

The Pathway of Peace

Shortly after we had returned from visiting Twylah on the Cattaraugus Reservation, we received a letter from her stating that she felt compelled to share with us the symbolic stepping stones and colors which the Seneca medicine people had used in the meditative exercise of going into the Silence. Properly practiced and rightfully employed as a psychical stimulus, the Pathway of Peace can lead one into the Great Silence, a spiritual ecstasy far beyond that of ordinary meditation.

Twylah said that she had spent three days in the Silence, seeking an answer as to whether the technique should be shared at this time. She interpreted all the symbols which came to her as positive assertions that the time was now, and that both Indians and non-Indians were mature enough to receive the lesson and the prayers and she should employ them in a respectful and fruitful manner.

She picked up a cassette tape on which to record the Pathway of Peace to mail to us for transcription. It was not until she had completed an initial taping that she realized she had recorded over a tape of her mother's voice. She played the tape through, reflecting on the words she had recorded, and sat for a few moments in pensive silence. Should she have released this material, she wondered. As if in answer to her unspoken question, she was startled to hear her mother's recorded voice saying, "It is good. It is good."

Herewith is *The Pathway of Peace*, a revelation shared by Twylah Hurd Nitsch:

The Pathway of Peace leads toward peace of mind
The sharing of gifts to every kind
Of creation living upon this earth,
Measuring the steps of each ones' worth.

Seek the trail of Seven Stones
Where Spiritual songs of harmonic tones
Fill the world in harmony,
Soothing throngs of creatures into serenity.

Desire peaks into the soul
Where gifts of life are there to behold
Where charms of peace and harmony
Belong to all for eternity.

"We are born into a limited human body into the material world. The search begins for self-knowledge to understand the environment that has so much influence on our personal lifestyle and personal development. We blend this knowledge to create principles that will guide our material existence. When spiritual awareness filters into our deeper senses, we secure peace and understanding, which highlights our personal lifestyle by permitting us to follow the universal laws and to become attuned with all creation.

"This spiritual unfoldment creates a person who lives a life of patience and understanding, who adheres to attitudes that govern his very existence. It shows in the example he lives and his ability to expel fear from his life.

"The early Seneca did this by going into the Silence, which followed four steps. The first was the purpose; the second, the preparation; the third, the procedure; the fourth, the progression.

"The purpose is to establish a personal routine for entering into the Silence that will become a regular experience in spiritual enrichment in one's lifestyle.

"The preparation is arranged for this solitary ritual as one would prepare for his daily intake of food, in order to satisfy the hunger for spiritual growth. We think of it as the spiritual nourishment that furnishes the lifeline, as well as the guideline, for our very existence. By preparing in this way, we can secure greater success.

"The procedure is to open the way for the spiritual forces to enter within the physical body through self-awareness. The procedure is called "Rekindling the Spiritual Light."

"There comes a time in everyone's life when becoming a seeker draws the individual closer to the spiritual self. The Seneca call this "approaching the first stone," or the "pathway of self-knowledge."

"Seven stepping stones mark the trail that leads the seeker into the Great Silence.

"*The first stepping stone,* the Blood-stone, glows in radiant shades of red. It plants the seed that awakens the seeker to the spiritual way of faith and beckons the seeker to the entrance of the Pathway of Peace.

"The Blood-stone has seven facets. Each facet designates one of the spiritual senses of sound, sight, scent, taste, touch, awareness, and emotions. Standing upon the first stone is symbolic of the life materialized in the physical world and is a daily venture in faith.

"The seeker learns that the Great Mystery, the Spiritual Essence, is connected with all things in creation and that all things in creation are connected with one another. It is the impressions influenced by this interconnection that affect the experiences in all creation.

"The radiance of the Blood-stone flows throughout the seeker and into the material world, uniting all creation into thoughts and feelings of faith.

"Becoming aware of the existence of the first stepping stone and the lessons it imparts opens the way to the second stepping stone on the Pathway of Peace.

"*The second stepping stone,* the Sun-stone, glows in radiant shades of yellow. It plants the seed that awakens the seeker to the spiritual way of love, and it beckons the seeker to dwell upon the Sun-stone on the Pathway of Peace.

"The Sun-stone has the same seven facets that designate the powerful spiritual senses of sound, sight, scent, taste, touch, awareness, and emotions. Standing upon the Sun-stone is symbolic of the life materialized in the physical world and is a daily venture in love.

"Its radiance of love flows throughout the seeker and into the material world. Faith and love go hand in hand. It is the spiritual expression of faith and love that makes the world go around and helps the seeker to grow in peace and harmony.

"Becoming aware of the existence of the Sun-stone and the lessons it imparts opens the way to the third stepping stone on the Pathway of Peace.

"*The third stepping stone,* the Water-stone, glows in radiant shades of blue. It plants the seed that awakens the seeker to the spiritual way of cleansing and soothing, and it beckons the seeker to dwell upon the Water-stone.

"The Water-stone has seven facets. Each facet designates one of the spiritual senses of sound, sight, scent, taste, touch, awareness, and emotions.

"Standing upon the Water-stone is symbolic of the life materialized in the material world and is a daily venture of cleansing and being soothed.

"The radiance of the Water-stone flows throughout the seeker and into the material world, nourishing it with cleansing purity. It is the fluid property that unites all creation into the stream of spirituality and helps the seeker grow toward peace and harmony through its expression of peaceful relaxation.

"Becoming aware of the existence of the Water-stone and the lessons it imparts opens the way to the fourth stepping stone on the Pathway of Peace.

"*The fourth stepping stone,* the Fertility-stone, glows in radiant shades of green. It plants the seed that awakens the seeker to the spiritual way of abundance and renewal, and it beckons the seeker to dwell upon the Fertility-stone.

"The Fertility-stone has seven sides, each designating one of the spiritual senses of sound, sight, scent, taste, touch, awareness, and emotions.

"Standing upon the Fertility-stone is symbolic of the life materialized in the material world and is a daily venture in physical and natural growth. Its radiance flows throughout the seeker and into the material world, nourishing it with abundant life.

"It is the renewing property of the fourth stepping stone that unites all creation into environmental awareness and helps the seeker grow toward peace and harmony.

"Becoming aware of the existence of the Fertility-stone and the lessons it imparts opens the way to the fifth stepping stone on the Pathway of Peace.

"*The fifth stepping stone,* the Blossoming-stone, glows in radiant shades of coral pink. It plants the seeds that awaken the seeker to the spiritual way of upliftment, and it beckons the seeker to dwell upon the fifth stepping stone on the Pathway of Peace. The Blossoming-stone has the same powerful facets as the previous stepping stones.

"The radiance of its unfolding properties flow throughout the seeker and into the material world, nourishing it with beauty and spiritual insight.

"Standing upon the Blossoming-stone is symbolic of the life materialized in the physical world. It offers a daily venture in intuitive impulses and is a gift received on the Pathway of Peace.

"Its properties of upliftment help the seeker grow toward peace and harmony.

"Becoming aware of the existence of the Blossoming-stone and the lessons it imparts opens the way to the sixth stone on the Pathway of Peace.

"*The sixth stepping stone,* the Charity-stone, glows in a radiant burst of spiritual light. It plants the seed that awakens the seeker to the spiritual way of benevolence in thoughts and deeds, and it beckons the seeker to dwell upon the sixth stepping stone on the Pathway of Peace.

"The Charity-stone has the same powerful facets as the stepping stones that preceded it.

"The radiance of the Charity-stone flows throughout the seeker and into the material world, nourishing it with acts of kindness and understanding.

"It is the charitable properties of the sixth stepping stone that unite all creation into the ways of Spiritual Harmony. Its brilliance crystallizes the highest spiritual self in preparation for entering into the Great Silence.

"Becoming aware of the sixth stepping stone and the lessons it imparts opens the way to the seventh stepping stone on the Pathway of Peace.

"*The seventh stepping stone,* the Healing-stone, glows in radiant shades of lavender. It plants the seed that awakens the seeker to the spiritual way of healing—the highest creative spirituality. It beckons the seeker to dwell on the seventh stepping stone on the Pathway of Peace.

"The radiance of the Healing-stone projects the powerful facets in sound, in sight, in scent, in taste, in touch, in awareness, and in emotions, and it flows into the seeker and into the material world, nourishing all creation with the Essence of Spiritual Healing that leads toward peace and harmony.

"The healing properties unite all creation into spiritual attunement, which flows throughout Eternity.

"Becoming aware of the existence of the seventh stepping stone leads to the threshold of the Great Silence that opens the way of Spiritual Peace and Harmony."

In the Silence
All creation unites and communicates
The Spiritual Way.
Where life is pure, life is fulfilling;
Life is understanding; life is sharing;
Life is abundant; life is unity; and
Life is Eternity.
The ecstasy of Spiritual Enlightenment.

As the seeker descends the Pathway of Peace—

The seventh stepping stone reveals Spiritual Healing.
The sixth stepping stone reveals Spiritual Charity.
The fifth stepping stone reveals Spiritual Insight.
The fourth stepping stone reveals Spiritual Awareness.
The third stepping stone reveals Spiritual Cleansing.
The second stepping stone reveals Spiritual Love.
The first stepping stone reveals Spiritual Faith.

The Light of all Light,
The Light of all Faith and Love,
The Light of all Knowledge and Inspiration,
The Source of all Creation—
The Spiritual Revelation.

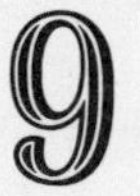

Archaeology and Anguish

> Clarkston, Washington (UPI)—Thieves invaded a 100-year-old Nez Perce Indian burial ground near here, stealing skulls and jewelry, anthropologists reported.
>
> Authorities said human skulls were worth $25 each and more in a bizarre underground market centered in California.
>
> "It makes me mad to just be around the place and see what has been done," said Richard Halfmoon of Lapwai, Idaho, chairman of the Nez Tribal Council. "They don't let our Indians rest in peace whether they are dead or alive.
>
> "We know the name of the dentist who has Chief Joseph's skull and uses it for an ashtray."
>
> Chief Joseph, the Nez Perce's greatest chief, was pursued by the U.S. Cavalry in the late 1800s when he led part of his tribe on a 1,500-mile escape to Canada.

"The time has come when we are wanting museums and everyone to return these [skeletal remains] so we can put them back in the proper place where they belong," commented Rolling Thunder, a Shoshone medicine man, who is regarded as one of the most influential of today's medicine people.

Cautious and respectful archaeologists and anthropologists are arranging ceremonies to be held over the excavation sites before a single shovel begins to turn over sacred soil.

Although technical supervision was provided by John Sigstead, curator of anthropology at the University of South Dakota, Vermillion, all of the work on the burial mound recently found west of Wilmot was done by Indians under the direction of the Sisseton–Wahpeton Sioux Tribal Council. In addition, according to Ed Red Owl of the Tribal Office, a medicine man performed a ceremony at the mound site in order to protect the workers and to maintain the dignity of the dead who were buried there. "We didn't want the excavation to be a sacrilege to the people buried there," Red Owl said.

Even though ceremonies and dead feasts are being conducted over sites where archaeological students are preparing to dig for skeletal clues to the Amerindian's past, there still remains the principal point of contention in many a serious Native American's mind that sacred ground is being desecrated. How complete must a ceremony be to compensate the grandfathers and grandmothers for defilement? Anthropological and archaeological violation of the final resting places of countless American Indian men, women, and children has not only set an ethnic pot to boiling, but scholarly shovels may have set in motion a series of psychic disturbances totally beyond their scientific ken.

"To us, the ashes of our ancestors are sacred and their resting place is hallowed ground," Chief Seattle told Governor Isaac Stevens when he surrendered his land in 1855.

Chief Joseph of the Nez Perce (that same noble warrior whose skull now serves as an ashtray in a dentist's office) was told by his own father: "My son, never forget my dying words. This country holds your father's body. Never sell the bones of your father and your mother."

Chief Joseph observed with fervor that "a man who would not love his father's grave is worse than a wild animal."

Museums, archaeologists, and anthropologists throughout the United States are discovering that there are numerous, and very vocal, Native Americans who do, indeed, love their fathers' graves.

Charles Ellenbaum, an anthropologist in charge of a dig at St. Charles, Illinois, conducted by the College of DuPage, resisted the arguments of the American Indian Center to cease his excavations. Mrs. Pat Rensch of the Indian Center told him, "If you people want to dig graves, dig up your own."

Ellenbaum countered by stating that the remains belonged to the owner of the dig site and that his studies would yield valuable information about the early American Indians of the Fox River Valley.

Susan Powers, chairman of the Board of Directors of the Indian Center, replied that Ellenbaum knew it was wrong to continue with the excavation. "The white man better start studying [himself]," she said. "Your world is falling apart. Your children are running away from you. You are a confused people."

Matthew War Bonnet, a Sioux and an instructor in Native American history at the Circle campus of the University of Illinois, led a protest group to the Field Museum of Natural History when spokesmen for the museum announced thier recent acquisition of the skeletal remains of nine Miami Indians, circa late seventeenth century. In response to War Bonnet's objections, curator Dr. Donald Collier issued a statement pointing out that the museum had always endeavored to treat the ancient dead with respect. The Field Museum would, Dr. Collier said, replace the bones and pay for any costs incurred. After an evening ceremonial fire officiated over by a medicine man, the museum delivered the remains to a Winnebago burial ground near the Wisconsin Dells.

When Mohawk Chief Lawrence Lazore learned that an archaeology professor and eighteen of his students had disinterred six skeletons from a burial ground near the St. Lawrence River in July 1972, he denounced the field trip as "plain grave robbery." Lazore, who presides over the St. Regis Reservation and who has an archaeology degree of his own, said that if archaeologists ". . . want to use cemeteries as laboratories for their students, they should use their own cemeteries."

In October 1972, Cherokee leaders protested against what they termed the plundering of ancestral graves by artifact-hunting archaeologists. The archaeologists defended their position by stating that they were rushing to uncover and preserve relics that will be lost forever when a Tennessee Valley Authority dam floods them in a few years.

Vice Chief John Crowe of the eastern band of Cherokees said that the TVA was going to flood ". . . a whole race of people's history and heritage off the map."

A TVA spokesman issued a statement declaring that they were funding the digging of Dr. Alfred K. Guthe, director of the McClung Museum at the University of Tennessee at Knoxville, so that the heritage to be found in the old Cherokee village and fort near Tellico Plains would not be destroyed.

The essential issue of whether to dig or not can be evaded by pointing a desperate finger toward progress. "Why not excavate Indian graves?" the archaeologist can shrug. "If we don't get the bones, the bulldozers and housing developments will."

Although it is difficult, try to visualize a Native American archaeologist descending upon some forgotten pioneer cemetery with his students and announcing his plans to excavate. "We wish to make an analysis of pioneer pathology," he might tell the press. "We are curious to see what diseases the early Anglos suffered in this area and how their pathology fits in with the larger frontier pattern. We are also curious to discover what artifacts these settlers buried with their dead, and we shall seek to determine what we can about the Anglo historical process from these relics."

What hue and cry would white America raise over such desecration? Or are the two situations analogous? An anthropologist could protest that the white settlers kept written records. We really know very little about early red America. Even the question of Native American origin is far from resolved. European physical traits are as strongly represented among the aboriginal tribes as Mongolian.

Just a few decades ago, the majority of textbooks taught that man did not arrive in the Americas until some adventurous Asiatics trudged across the Bering land bridge at about the time of Christ. Certain anthropologists were prepared to state that man may have been in the New World by 3,000 B.C. but only a few academic anthropologists and archaeologists were foolhardy enough to suggest that man may have been in the Americas as early as 8,000 B.C. Then in 1952, Dr. Paul Sears of Yale University dug up some maize pollen grain from about 240 feet below the surface of the dried lake bed on which Mexico City is built.

Maize is the most highly developed agricultural plant in the world, so highly developed that scientists have never been able to trace it back to its original ancestors. According to radiocarbon testing, the pollen grains from the Mexican lake bed are at least 25,000 years old.

In 1960, Dr. Juan Armente Comacho, director of the Department of Anthropology at the University of Puebla in Mexico, dug a piece of a mastodon's pelvic bone out of the desert soil at Balsequello, sixty miles southeast of Mexico City. On the bone's surface, some ancient artist had engraved the images of a horse, a camel, a reptile, and a type of mastodon thought to have been extinct for 100,000 years.

Dr. H. Marie Wormington, curator of archaeology at the Denver Museum of Natural History, stated that the artwork and the bone were contemporary. The carving could only have been done on fresh bone, Dr. Wormington said, not fossil bone.

Certain authorities believe that the earliest immigrants to arrive in the Americas via the Bering Strait were definitely Europid-Caucasian in type. In their opinion, the Mongol migrations probably did not occur until 2,000 B.C., and then from the Pacific as well as Siberia.

"It is because of this very late admixture of yellow blood that the various tribes of America create a Mongoloid impression, which has given rise to their erroneous classification in the Mongol race," stated the German ethnologist Ivar Lissner. "For many tens of thousands of years the early inhabitants of American were the descendants of paleo-Europid peoples who had also occupied Siberia."

When the Europeans began their invasion of North America early in the sixteenth century there were about three hundred different tribes with a combined population of over one million. Today with a population of about 800,000, the Native American is far from a vanishing race, and, although some tribes have been totally decimated, others, such as the Navajo, the Sioux, and the Cherokee have grown in numbers.

The serious anthropologist does not regard him- or herself as a grave robber. Quite the contrary, s/he conceptualizes him- or herself as a guardian of Indian culture who is working in basically the same direction as the Indian. At the same time, s/he recognizes the fact that s/he must walk a thin line between two cultures and deal with a situation in which the anthropologist and the archaeologist are perceived as the enemy. Anthropologist R. Clark Mallam agreed to talk with me about how it feels to have the shoe of prejudice now on the other foot.

R. Clark Mallam: "The American Indian today is an individual who is becoming aware of his heritage; and as he becomes aware of his heritage, he also becomes aware of his identity. Since he is an individual who possesses a distinct identity, it is logical, then, that anything that is held in a museum is considered denigrative to that identity. If I were curator of a museum, I would state that the displays of artifacts are not denigrative to the Indian people. The displays are there for the purpose of preserving that particular cultural aspect which would be lost, given the location of most of these burial grounds.

"By and large, judging from where most of these Indian cemeteries or mounds have been located in the past, it is logical to assume that, as some archaeologists have suggested, within the next fifty years there is hardly going to be an Indian site in America that will be worth studying, because of our rapid mobility in terms of building urban and suburban areas. In areas where Indian burial grounds are not located on reservations, the graves are open to vandalism and to commercial exploitation of the grossest sort. At the same time, they are open to real estate dealers who can sell the land and permit the artifacts to be simply bulldozed away and scattered.

"I think we are dealing with a situation in which there are levels of denigration. These so-called artifacts—especially human artifacts—are of immense value in reconstructing a prehistoric cultural history of the

American Indian. From these skeletal remains, we can learn how long the Indian has lived, what diseases he was susceptible to, and a variety of other important populational and demographic factors."

How can such information be important and helpful to the American Indian of today?

Mallam: "I think in some cases the Indian does not realize the potentiality of how he can be helped by this information. At the same time, many anthropologists and archaeologists have reduced this information to an inner circle of discussion, and they have not been taking this information and disseminating it to the American public so that some of the stereotypes and myths that are so rampant in white culture regarding the Indian might be eliminated.

"In my opinion, we in American archaeology are, in terms of our dealing with the American Indians, at an impasse, an impasse that has been prompted by the archaeologist's inability to accept the fact that his information is of sufficient use that it can be disseminated to the public and have a practical value associated with it. The archaeologist's failure to recognize this has resulted in the Indian stating that his services are derogatory to Indian identity.

"If the artifacts are to be kept within a closed circle of academicians, then I favor their being restored to the rightful owners.

"I would say that we are dealing with a series of social processes in which individuals of different identities are motivated and actuated by different things. The archaeologist makes his bread and his name by discovering a site, working it, publishing it, and ultimately having artifacts from it displayed somewhere. From that type of research, the archaeologist will achieve a certain degree of fame and, at the same time, will be recognized by his college and by his particular department, thereby giving him rank, perhaps tenure, and greater accessibility to funds for future work. Indian artifacts are, in this sense, a prime means for an individual in the field of archaeology to achieve status in his society.

"Now, this system is completely antithetical to the Indian concept of obtaining status, because the artifacts are limited and there is competition for the obtaining of the artifacts. Competition is a term that is not really known to the American Indian. If you were to draw a very generalized picture of the world view of American Indians, it would be one of cooperation and harmony. The Indian cannot see what moves the white archaeologists, and the white archaeologists cannot see what moves the Indian, so we are at an impasse.

"What we need is compromise, and the compromise has to be worked out within the context of the situation in which it occurs. I don't believe we can legislate anything dealing with artifacts. I don't think it is possible to legislate a morality borne between two cultures. We will have to have people of understanding on both sides."

What if a process of understanding with a living culture had started one hundred fifty years ago?

Mallam: "It did almost start one hundred fifty years ago with Thomas Jefferson directing the archaeological excavation of some mounds."

But then progress and Manifest Destiny and the westward movement would not be denied.

Mallam: "Right. I have been doing some research on the history of the mound-builder myth. Because of the assumptions that whites had about this New World, the mounds were not really ascribed to Indian creation until about 1890. It is interesting that the actual death of the mound-builder myth tends to coincide in a general fashion with the massacre at Wounded Knee in 1892, which was the last major confrontation between whites and Indians. And 1890 is also the official closing of the frontier for the U.S. Bureau of Census. What we are saying is that it was impossible one hundred fifty, or even one hundred years ago, for the whiteman to have had this type of interest in the Indian, because people were acting upon sets of cultural assumptions that were logical and positive to them at that time."

What if there had been a controlled immigration program that slowed up the western movement considerably. Could this have encouraged greater interaction and understanding between the two cultures?

Mallam: "It might have worked; but, you see, the Indian never had a chance once white contact was made, because white contact spread so rapidly that there was a great deal of acculturation going on between Indians and whites from the very onset. Indians recognized that whites had certain cultural traits that were of value to them; so, they took them and incorporated them into their own society. Whites did the same thing. In fact, almost any meal we eat today is largely derived from Indian foods that were produced independently on this continent.

"But if there had been no pressure to settle the New World, and if there had been controlled immigration to the New World, then the situation might have changed so that the Indians would have at least achieved a status of purity in the interaction with whites. The Indians did have that status at the very beginning of colonization, even though there were basic cultural assumptions about their inferiority.

"Once the seaboard was occupied, however, and the penetrations had begun into the interior, a process was started whereby one Indian tribe was being moved out until it came into contact with another Indian tribe, and a snowball effect was created. There was constant pressure on the Indian to preserve his own lifestyle in the face of an encroaching civilization.

"Under circumstances of acculturation whereby two sides view themselves as complete, politically autonomous units, there is an excellent chance for understanding. But the political autonomy of the Indian soon began to disappear, and he became the victim of a whole series of programs directed toward the very base of his existence, which is his identity."

Once you have obtained the proper legal permissions, do you feel any qualms in unearthing bones from a burial mound? Would you feel that you were desecrating sacred ground?

Mallam: "Specifically, I, as an individual, would be fully aware that the mound was a sacred place, but I am faced with a situation where it is almost an either/or situation in the sense that either someone who is trained and knowledgeable about Indian mythology and history can handle these artifacts with discretion, or the relics can be left alone and eventually be rooted out by vandals. I cannot think of one mound in the state of Iowa—with the exception of the Effigy Mounds National Monument—that has not been potted by vandals. These are the artifacts that find their way into private collections and are displayed on mantelpieces."

You advise making pragmatic use of a deplorable situation.

Mallam: "I think you can say I advise making pragmatic use of a deplorable situation in the hope that, ultimately, the end result will be aesthetic and that there will be a new understanding created.

"What I am trying to do here in northeast Iowa is to write a history of Indians from prehistoric times to the present which can be utilized in the classrooms of grades one through six. The idea is that the archaeological work that we conduct in northeast Iowa will be used for illustrating Indian identity and will be disseminated directly to the elementary school as a specific part of social studies units which deal with American Indians.

"I feel that if factual and valid information is presented to children at the elementary level, proper Indian/white structural relationships can be created. From what I have seen, most of the material that comes out of the American public school system, at least in the elementary grades, is so ethnocentric and degrading that the child builds up a set of cultural assumptions that will permit him to see no wrong in destroying Indian sites, because Indians are a thing of the past and are gone. If we are not pragmatic, we are going to watch a whole series of Indian sites and sacred places be destroyed."

Two Navajos and a Hopi recently filed suit in Coconino County Superior Court in an effort to halt a zoning decision that would permit a ski village to be constructed on the San Francisco Peaks north of Flagstaff, Arizona. According to the Indians, Navajo, Apache, Hopi, Camp Verde Yavapai, Havasupai, Walpi, and Pueblo people regard the area as holy.

Robert Lomadafkie, Jr., warned that the high winds and the continuing drought in the area were no accident. "The spirits are angry," he said, regarding the plans of Summit Properties, a Flagstaff development firm, to fashion ski jumps and chalets on the Sacred Western Mountain. To Lomadafkie, Jr., a Hopi, the Holy Mountain is the home of the Kachina spirit people.

Bill Beavor, operator of Sacred Mountain Trading Post, saw the central issue as being one that pitted skiers and business against Indians and religion. "You wouldn't ski through the Vatican," he said. "You wouldn't throw snowballs in the Tabernacle in Salt Lake City. That's basically what it boils down to."

For the traditional American Indian, there is a very thin line of demarcation between the living and the dead. As Chief Seattle remarked, "There is no death, only a change of worlds." A major portion of traditional Indian medicine is the deep and abiding belief in personal contact with the unseen world of the grandmothers and grandfathers. This medicine suggests that direct communication with this invisible world is possible, and that the dead and the living depend upon one another in countless ways which fashion and uphold the world.

As Don Wanatee, a Mesquakie, told me:

> We have maintained the basic ways of our ancestors, so therefore we are in direct contact with them every day. As a matter of fact, the beliefs that we practice today are basically for them, because we believe that the dead take care of the living, as the living take care of the dead.

10
Spiritual Warrior of the Sioux

"A cowboy and an Indian die and go to heaven. They get met by St. Peter at the pearly gates, and St. Pete ushers the cowboy into a Cadillac. The angels come out and they line the streets. They start to cheer and the cowboy is driven down between the rows of angels while they stand there applauding and tossing confetti, ticker tape, streamers. The Indian is given an old Model-T that can just barely sputter. By the time the old clunker reaches the parade route, nearly all the angels have gone home.

"The Indian is a little upset. 'I had to take all that abuse on earth, he grumbles. 'Now when I go to heaven, I get the same treatment. The cowboy is up front in the Cadillac, and I'm in the back in an old Model-T.'

"St. Peter takes the Indian aside, puts an arm around him, and says, 'You must understand. We are pleased to have you in heaven, but, you see, this is the first cowboy we've ever had!"

With a unique teaching technique, Dallas Chief Eagle uses humor to transform hurt and pain. When Chief Eagle takes the old "cowboy-and-Indian" motif so familiar to anyone who has grown up in a nation of Saturday matinées, cap pistols, and Manifest Destiny and combines it with the whiteman's religious hope of a reward on the "other side," he manages to take two of the dominant culture's cherished symbols and turn them around to make a joke on the whiteman.

Humor also permits Chief Eagle to juxtapose past and present and to offer guidance for the future.

"There was this time when I was supposed to speak on this campus. When I arrived, I found it embroiled in the protests of activist students.

And here I am supposed to speak about the redman and his problems. I decided to change my lecture format, and I called right away for questions from the audience.

"Right away, a young woman asks, 'What do you think about the invasion of Cambodia? Do you think the United States will continue its invasion, or do you think that the U.S. will stop, as it has promised?'

"I answered, 'Miss, I think the United States will be like the rapist who says, "Don't worry, ma'am. I'll just go in an inch!" ' "

Each Indian nation is all too familiar with this approach, as in treaty violation after treaty violation, the whiteman told the Indian, "Don't worry. We're just going to take a little bit more of your land."

Dallas Chief Eagle does not live in the buffalo-hide teepees of his Lakota (Sioux) ancestors. He lives with his family in a small, modest home in Pierre, South Dakota. His life is now in the city, where he is director of tourism for the Development Corporation of the United Sioux Tribes of South Dakota. His wife Shirley, a Brule Sioux, together with the daughters still at home, offer Dallas Chief Eagle both a happy home life and the inspiration to gain the most advantages from the system that he can for his people.

The Chief Eagle residence, just two blocks off the end of main street, is a comfortable, inviting home. Kids and their friends sprawl in front of after-school television. A statue of the Virgin Mary stands on a mirrored cabinet. A large drum rests in a corner of the dining room. Medicine articles and Chief Eagle's own inspired medicine paintings hang about the house. Like its owner, the home reflects a blending of traditional Native American culture and Medicine Power with twentieth-century, middle-American aspirations.

Many years ago, Dallas Chief Eagle made a promise to himself that he would write a book about the Sioux that would be as culturally authentic and as historically accurate as he could make it. In 1967 *Winter Count* (Johnson Publishing, Boulder, Colorado) appeared. Chief Eagle wrote the book six times in four years, working at night after he had completed his regular shift at a steel mill. In addition to his credit as a novelist, Chief Eagle is also an accomplished painter who specializes in American Indian scenes.

In a special ceremony held in October 1967 the Teton Sioux elected Dallas Bordeaux their chief. The great chief Red Cloud was named to the title in 1868, and when he died his people chose not to select a new chief out of respect to the wise leader and skilled military strategist.

Chief Red Cloud defeated the United States troops in every major encounter and won all the treaty concessions he demanded. To succeed Red Cloud is a great honor.

A feast and a powwow were held, and Chief Eagle was presented with Red Cloud's pipe, which bears 112 notches on it for the number of Indians, soldiers, and settlers personally killed by the war chief during his lifetime. A number of Indians cited Chief Eagle's past accomplishments, including his novel *Winter Count*. A restricted number of elders were present at the ceremony: Edgar Red Cloud and Charlie Red Cloud sponsored Chief Eagle; the matron of honor was Alice Black Horse; and Ceremonial Chief Frank Fools Crow conferred the honor. The Bureau of Indian Affairs does not officially recognize Dallas Chief Eagle as chief of the Tetons, choosing, rather to regard the title as honorary.

Since Chief Eagle's wife Shirley is descended from the famous Brule chief Spotted Tail, it should hardly be surprising to learn that they decided long ago to rear their children in a combination of modern, midstream North American culture and American Indian traditionalism. At the same time that he is a devout student of nature according to the ancient tribal philosophy, Dallas Chief Eagle is also a practicing Roman Catholic. Chief Eagle believes in blending—in one practice and philosophy drawing from another.

"I have delved deeply into the ways of my ancestors," he said. "I know that there is great wisdom and good in Indian theology. I have never believed that Christianity has a franchise on religion. Wisdom is God-given, and you can get it only through the study of nature.

"So it is in the material aspects of life. In order to generate interest in the products of the American Indian, we have to use the whiteman's method of promotion. White technology should be applied to producing Indian goods. We need both cultures. We should not try to destroy one another. We do not have to merge or integrate, but we can learn to take the good from each and apply it to our modern life."

What would be the most common symbol for the Great Spirit among the Lakota?

Dallas Chief Eagle: "There is no symbol as such for the Great Spirit. The closest would be the symbol of peace, the pipe or the crossed pipes, with the stem upward."

Would wakan *be the best word in Lakota for the Great Mystery?*

"Wakan means holy, sacred."

Some authorities say that wakan is the word for the Great Spirit, but it seems that the translation of "Great Mystery" or "an essence that permeates all life" would be better.

"Yes, because the Indian never sat around trying to figure out what the Great Spirit looked like.

"We pay homage to this Great Spirit, or Great Mystery, through his own creations—the Sun, the Earth, the wind, the thunder, the lightning. The earth must not be spoiled by the men who worship in mere lodges, by the arrogance of those who have never known defeat, by the self-righteousness of those who violate treaties and punish those who would resist such violations.

"As we stand uneasily in the border country of the Atomic Age, we have set our feet on spiritual pathways which may thrust us against furies of nature and man which can overpower us as unsympathetically as the blue-coated cavalry overpowered the Sioux. Instead of courage and determination, we have developed productivity and comfort. These may be our undoing. Whether one lives as a Sioux or a middle-class American, he can find his highest ideals subverted to savagery and greed.

"The Great Mystery made nature for us to use and preserve; but, nature also imposes obligations upon us. We are only passing through life on our way to the Spirit World of our ancestors.

"We Indians must pray to the Holy Mystery and ask that some day the whitemen will better understand us, that the needs of their consciousness will awake and grow. Our freedom is our way of life, but to others, it could be a different thing. You have to know what you are in order to feel the Great Spirit in nature. It is only through nature that one can gain communion with the Holy Mystery."

You have expressed so much of yourself and your heritage in Winter Count. *Are you able to utilize your paintings in the same dual role of self-expression and teaching?*

"I think so. The early Indian sensed the beauty of nature and expressed it in art. My forefathers made storytelling pictographs, which led to abbreviated picture-writing. Some present-day artists use a conglomeration of abbreviated pictures combined into one scope and tab it modern art. I am certain my ancestors would disagree violently with this kind of painting.

"As an Indian artist, I seek to express myself through the past and through tradition, which is interwoven with Indian theology. The early Indian artists who worked with crude tools and simple pigments left proof that great art does not necessarily relate to the so-called intellectual attainments of civilization. Great art rises from basic human emotions and is timeless.

"In my opinion, modern abstract art is immoral. It is a selfish restriction of a God-given resource. It is a camouflage. It is like putting a cloak over something that would otherwise be beautiful."

Chief Eagle, let us talk about your personal background. You know, all the vital statistics.

"I was born in 1925 in a tent on the Rosebud Reservation. That tent wasn't an Indian teepee; it was a Montgomery Ward tent. I was orphaned as a child, and, according to our culture, the eldest of the tribe are to raise the orphans.

"Those who brought me up taught me not to accept the non-Indian ways of life. They would not even let me learn English. To them, everything was temporary. Such a belief can be traced back to their history. The Lakota were nomads. They never had a permanent place to live. Even if some marauding tribe were to conquer them, this would be only a temporary condition. So when the big European invasion came, they regarded it as a temporary condition. They knew the old ways would come back. This is why they taught me that it was useless to learn the whiteman's lifestyle.

"I had quite an experience on my first day of school. I reluctantly went with the agency police and a Jesuit missionary to the mission school."

Why were the police there?

"To make certain that I stayed in school! I was five, six years old. I didn't speak English; I knew only Sioux people.

"Anyway, my experience came with the language. A nun was teaching us English, and I couldn't understand a word she was saying. I couldn't respond to anything she said. She finally grabbed me by the elbows and stood me up in the middle of the aisle. She jabbered some more, took me by the arm, and led me to a corner, where she set me on a stool and put a long, pointed cap on my head.

"I was a very proud little boy. The way I had been raised had conditioned me to accept that any type of commendation, any type of decoration, any honor would be conferred on the head. I thought to myself, here it is my first day at the whiteman's school, and already I have been recognized as a superior little boy. I have been given a fine headdress.

"Then, at recess time, my classmates told me that I was wearing a dunce cap. I was being punished for not being able to speak English."

I suppose most whites would be surprised to learn that many Indian children on the reservations do not speak English until they are exposed to the public, or mission, schools. How many Indians would you say are bilingual?

"In this last half of the twentieth century, I would say about one-fourth are bilingual. In my opinion, this is very unfortunate. There is a great deal of knowledge to be gained from the Indian language.

"Wisdom does not come from institutions. It comes from a higher power. We do not identify this higher power as a human being. We do not identify it as any one particular energy or life. The higher power, the Great Mystery, is identified by all energies in life. The Great Mystery is in a blade of grass, an animal, a fowl, the thunder, or a rock.

"Most of the Sioux west of the Missouri are Tetons, which comprises over three-fourths of the Sioux tribes. We use the 'l' not the 'd' when we speak. Lakota not Dakota. I fear our young people are losing a great deal of their culture and their heritage. They don't try to learn Indian from their elders. I think this is a great loss to America and to the system.

How would you compare English and Lakota in terms of effectiveness of communication?

"I have never really given this much thought. I would say that Russian would be fairly easy for a Lakotan to learn because of their pronunciations. In my trips to Japan I have found that many of their words have the same pronunciations, but entirely different meanings.

"I have always been quite amazed by the fact that the Jews called God 'Jahweh.' I think of the Passover, of the Jews bloodying the doorposts. In Sioux, Jahweh means 'to make the levy.'

"When I joined the United States Marines in 1942, I had to fill out a questionnaire. It asked, 'What foreign language do you speak?' I put down 'English.' The Marine Corps papers made a big thing of it, but I was serious."

Was the school you attended a boarding school?

"Yes."

What do you think it does to Indian kids to be educated in that kind of environment?

"I think it is complete isolation. I didn't get used to it until I was fourteen years old. If you want to look at things from a humane point of view, the reservations themselves are really set up as stockades. Boarding school was just a little step from the stockade environment into restrictiveness. Boarding schools take you away from people. I don't think this is very educational.

"They have changed the system since then, and I am very glad. Even though an Indian child may not know a word of English until he comes to school, his IQ is equal to that of any other American child. When an Indian child goes to school, however, right around fourth or fifth grade, he begins to realize that he is a very different person."

What causes that realization?

"The things that he is taught have no relevance to his way of life. There is nothing in the textbooks about the great chiefs, the great warriors, or the spiritual principles of Indianness. And the books talk about dad going to work in a taxi, getting in an elevator, and being taken to his executive offices in a skyscraper. This way of life has no relevance to the Indian child. These things are phenomenal to him."

Why does it take until the fourth or fifth grades for this realization to occur?

"That is the way the curriculum is set up. Before those grades, the Indian kid thinks, 'I am just a kid like these other guys.' But then the teachings of the whiteman start to show him that he is out of the circle. He begins to lose his sense of belonging. He starts looking around him, and he sees everything—the teacher, his classmates, even the movies he sees—telling him that he is a different kind of person."

Then in about the fifth grade he starts reading in his history book how the great heroes and military leaders of the last century did their best to solve the terrible Indian problem for the United States by annihilating as many tribes as possible.

"Right then the Indian kid realizes, 'Hey, these people are really down on me!' He gets this feeling of being dispossessed. Maybe a year or two later this psychological depression and alienation builds in him to the breaking point. Then we experience increased absenteeism. Maybe in seventh or eighth grade he drops out; maybe he waits until high school.

"The Indian child is confused. He believes that he doesn't belong. He knows only that the system regards him as an underling. He sees nothing which indicates that the system is interested in him or wants to help him. There is no way that a whiteman can really understand the psychological impact that reservation life can have on an Indian child.

"Let me give you an example. Let us say that the Communist Chinese come to where you live. They tell you that they have conquered the United States and that you are now their prisoner. You haven't got a thing to worry about, they say, because they have worked out an agreement, a treaty, between the Chinese people and the American people. The Chinese will now feed, clothe, and educate you. Pretty nice, huh? All your needs will be taken care of. Of course, you don't own anything now. The Chinese will confiscate your bank accounts, your cars, your homes.

"Then one day they say that your city is no longer to be your home. Chinese immigrants wish to settle there. You will be moved to an arid piece of land. Your home belongs to the Chinese. That miserable piece of land over there is yours.

"But again they tell you, don't worry. The land does not need to be green and fertile. They will feed you; they will clothe you; they will provide for your every need. But now they don't want you or your kids to speak English any more. You will speak only Chinese or you will be punished severely. And the clothes? From now on, it will be only Chinese-style pajama clothing. Food? No more meat and potatoes. From now on, rice and slivers of raw fish are what is good for you. And get rid of those knives and forks! Civilized people eat with chopsticks.

"Of course your children need to read and to write—Chinese. And the history books now emphasize the glories of the Chinese people, concentrating upon the period after the advent of Marxism in their country. White leaders are made to appear as buffoons and evil men.

"And your religious practices must go! No more of this brain-softening Christianity. Forget your religions and memorize the teachings of Chairman Mao."

I am getting the picture very vividly, Chief Eagle.

"Well, now you see that even though all your physical needs may be well provided for by another people, you can be left with nothing. Psychological destruction is one of the most terrible things that you can do to another human being."

Do you feel that reservations have been little more than prisoner-of-war camps?

"From the traditional Indian point of view, in a prisoner-of-war camp, you have hope. You know that someday the war will end. On the reservations there is no hope."

Is the school system on the Rosebud Reservation today more like that of mainstream American society?

"Right now it is moving that way. The missionary schools have been converted to day schools; there is no boarding school. In other South Dakota communities, there are Indians and non-Indians serving together on school boards, and the kids mix together. This gives them all a sense of belonging. It is a shame that it had to take a century for the whiteman to realize some of these things.

"Red Cloud himself wanted education for his people. He made several trips to Washington to plead for teachers. He received only negative responses until his last trip, when some Jesuits took notice of his plea. They established Holy Rose Mission, and even though about four years ago the name of the school was changed to Red Cloud Indian School, most Indians still refer to the institution as Holy Rose."

I hear so often of Indian youths involved in court cases because they have refused to cut their long, Indian-style hair.

"The long hair helps to build pride. You cannot motivate people until they have developed their sense of pride. These kids are desperately searching for identity. They figure that under the new civil rights rulings they can at least exercise the external appearance aspect of their traditionalism.

"These kids are learning to be active, and that is good in a democratic system. Activism makes the white people take notice. You have to take care of a squeak in the wheel, whether or not the noise comes from a minority. The whiteman founded this country on revolutionary tactics. I think the Indians taking over the offices of the Bureau of Indian Affairs in Washington is parallel to the Boston Tea Party. If you want to change this system, believe me, you have to use an ax to gain attention. That is the only way you can make this system readjust itself to become more responsive to those it governs."

Are there any other personal memories of your early educational experience that you would like to share?

"Well, yes, maybe it is time we had a smile.

"This same nun who grabbed me and punished me with a dunce cap because I did not know how to speak English always used to walk around the classroom with one of these metal frog clickers. You know what I mean? Those things you press with thumb and forefinger to make them go 'click-clack.'

"She would say, 'Class, put away your books [click-clack!].' 'Class [click-clack!], it is time for recess.' 'Class, pick up your pencils and papers and get back to work [click-clack!].' She really had us regimented. She was a very strict disciplinarian, yet we knew that she represented God on earth, in spite of that frog clicker in her hand.

"One day she gave us an assignment in art. We were to draw our conception of what God looked like. As I told you—and as you well know—such a project is totally alien to the Indian theology; but, we were learning to think like white children.

"I had my catechism on my desk, and it had a picture of Jesus on the cover. I figured that, since Jesus was the son of God, God must look like an older Jesus. So I used that as my model and handed in my assignment. I fared pretty well but the poor little girl next to me really got a scolding and got set in a corner. She drew a picture of God as a giant frog.

"Here is a poem that I have written about myself:

In an Indian tent he was born.
In a crowded school he was alone.
In a modern world his legs would bend.
Only on canvas and paper he lives his heritage.

"I think that gives a pretty good poetic word-picture of how I see myself. Here is another, more general, portrait of the Amerindian":

THE ROCKY MOUNTAIN INDIAN

The center of this land was my home,
A rainbow country flung high by the Great Spirit,
Where the earth meets the playground of clouds and
thunder.
Its highest peaks veiled with the haze of the starland,
Like teepees in the sky, fashioned by Spirit hands,
They loom as unchallenged monuments of earth.

None of the bow and arrow tell of this high empire,
Where the roving winds bow to its granite forms,
With lakes like random robes upon the council floor
Lay mirroring nature with peaceful meditation.
Reflected, too, are the frowning walls of jagged cliffs
Its heights held hostage to the turbulent streams.

Once forest tongues spoke in nature's dialect,
Where animals played in the hallowed realms of green,
Where the haunting calls of love-flutes made envy.
And tom-toms vibrated in the aspen plots, as dancing
black-haired children laughed and sang,
Their voices heard over the noisy foamed-rivers.

Then from the dawn country came the new noise of strife,
crushing the things of the spirit with alarm.
The land now echoed with shouts and curses of greed
The alien needs rang high in authority to destroy a creed
of ancient rights and legends.
The palefaces' hunt was on.

Werewolves began to split the stillness of the forest.
The air was choked with laws of different moods and minds;
The smoking mystery irons pushed down the tomahawks.
Anguished grief-chants condensed through the night.
Like the big freeze, icy resentment tortured the native man,
Leaving him little room to stand.
Famine began to stalk the teepees of the Rocky Mountains,
pushing scarred and unbowed heads to the flatlands.
Brute passion ruled the invaders' minds and hands.
A sad change came to the land of the Rockies.
Now only the solemn spruce stands wake over my ancestors.
The paleface came to stay.

What was your experience in the Marine Corps?

"I was in the Marine Corps from 1942 until I was discharged in October 1945. All I can say is that with General MacArthur's help, I won the war in the Southwest Pacific.

"You can check this out: The highest percentage of all the volunteers in World War I, World War II, Korea, and Vietnam came from the American Indians. I asked an aunt of mine which branch of service I should enter, and she said I would really look beautiful in a Marine Corps uniform. I was sad that she died when I was overseas, and she never did see me in my uniform.

"I filled one pocket with Indian bread—or 'cowboy bread' as non-Indians call it—and hitchhiked to Rapid City, the nearest place where I could join the Marine Corps. I spoke to this sergeant, and he gave me a bunch of papers. He told me to fill them out, and they would call me in a month or so. I told him that I didn't think I could live that long! So he put me up in a hotel that night and the following day he sent me off to Minneapolis to take my physical.

"The Marine Corps gave me some problems, but not like you would think. I was given some pretty tough assignments, because my superiors reasoned that, since I was an Indian, I would make a good scout.

" 'Go out there and track the enemy down,' they'd say, 'then shoot some tracer bullets at them so your squad will know where they are.'

"The trouble is, when you let these bullets go, the enemy knows where *you* are, too! I would shoot the tracers, then run like hell for another spot to crouch.

"Here were the good old stereotypes again. The officers took it for granted that I was the same caliber of warrior that my ancestors were."

Was it back to Rosebud after the war was over?

"I went back and finished my high school. Then I went to Chicago and took some specialized courses. I went to Oklahoma A&M and to Tulsa City College. I also attended the University of Idaho at Pocatello.

"I was a laborer for a long time. When I went to college, I was the best janitor on the job. I have been an industrial engineer and an industrial relations man for a steel corporation. I was a public relations man for H.L. Hunt for two years. I worked as a main negotiator for the United States Steel workers and as a financial secretary for them.

"After representing all those thousands of steel workers and their families, being their negotiator and agreements man, serving sometimes as their priest, I got to thinking about going back to my people and helping them. All my life I have felt that I had a role to fulfill. I still feel that I am not quite in my proper role. I know that I have a commitment that I can't quite identify as yet. The mystics, the Yuwipi people, tell me that a more important role is coming for me to fulfill."

Could that role be to devote yourself full time to medicine work?

"I do not know that I am worthy. Look at me; I smoke too much for one thing. I practice medicine, but there are so many administrative tasks that I feel I must do for my people.

"You know, Indian medicine, Indian theology, involves a great deal of what we now call parapsychology. Whenever I come to visit our holy men, they are always waiting for me. They always know when I will come.

"I have seen these holy men bathe their hands in liquid prepared from boiling herbs and be able to place their hands in flames with impunity. I have seen a wise man drink a tea for three days and be able to read my thoughts as specifically as I read a book. I have tried to jumble my thoughts and confuse him when he does this, but I have never succeeded in distracting him from accuracy."

For the present, then, it would seem that you consider yourself more activist than shaman.

"I am more of an activist now, that is true. But the Yuwipi men have asked me to develop the mystical part of my life more than I have."

Perhaps right now, you might be classified as a warrior-mystic, such as your ancestor Crazy Horse was.

"Yes, I am a mystic, but I must now fight for Indian causes. And I am definitely an activist. I feel, however, that one does not have to bend over toward radicalism or even revolutionary means. I think Dr. Martin Luther King with his example and his work did more for the Indians and other minority groups than Lincoln, Roosevelt, the Kennedys, or anyone."

Do you combine Roman Catholicism with traditional medicine power?

"I am more of a traditionalist, but I do live a bicultural existence.

"I like the term acculturation a lot better than assimilation or integration, because when you assimilate or integrate, you have to give up your Indianism. You have to take what the dominant society demands.

"I think I have mastered the art of bicultural livelihood. I think the educational institutions should take a closer look at what they are teaching and recognize that one does not have to give up his Indianism to learn how to master a livelihood acceptable to the dominant society.

"I could be 100 percent Indian, as far as culture is concerned. Tomorrow I could go down to the reservation and be 100 percent Indian. Today, I am sitting here with you like an average, middle-class man.

"I am bilingual; I am bicultural; and as far as my religion is concerned, I am also a 'bi.' My faith in Indian theology is equally as strong as my faith in Christianity. I rely on faith. I see a lot of things wrong with Christianity, but I can live with it. At the same time, I am not about to let a lot of my Indian religion go, because I value its principles higher than Christianity's dogmas and doctrines. I am 'bi,' and I feel absolutely no conflict at all."

There are a number of Native Americans who feel that they must go back to the ways their forefathers worshipped, that they must go back to the ways that the Great Spirit intended. Other Amerindians say that Apostolic Christianity—Christianity minus its multitude of dogmas—and Amerindian traditionalism are very close, and they see where it is possible for the two to blend. Would you agree with this?

"I certainly do. The movement of Christianity has become twisted because man has interjected too much into its spiritual flow. Dogmas! How can any man say what the Great Spirit thinks? The Supreme Power gives man a message, sets an example. The Great Mystery sets forth guidelines. If man puts forth any dogma or doctrine, I think he has put forth a challenge to the Great Spirit."

You would always hold your own visions above any dogma?

"Definitely, because that vision comes from the Great Spirit to me. I think it would be an insult to the Great Mystery to discard his message in favor of following one of his creation's dogmas."

Have you ever been accused of reinforcing white stereotypes of the Indian because you practice such "superstitions" as medicine power?

"Let those who mock medicine practice experience it. You know, we Indians were advanced in our social customs, as well as our spiritual expression when the Great Invasion came to our shores.

"The women of today are asking for equality. The American Indians had equality. Women served on our councils. Women played a very influential part in the affairs of a tribe, band, or clan. During the Great Invasion, the whitemen would not deal with our Indian women leaders. Even in the treaty affairs, they would not deal with our Indian women leaders. They excluded them from the meetings.

"The whiteman came and destroyed many things for us. The whiteman was in his puberty then. There still are not many who have matured."

Chief Eagle, you deal with the world on the terms demanded by the twentieth century, and it is obvious that you do not feel embarrassment practicing traditional medicine, nor do you regard yourself as a superstitious person.

"If I am superstitious, one would have to call Abraham, Moses, and Isaac superstitious. They all went on vision quests; so did Jesus. They all went into the wilderness to fast. Moses received the Ten Commandments on a vision quest. The Bible may not use that term, but the Biblical figures and the Indians practice the same procedure for the same purpose."

Do many Native Americans still embark on the vision quest?

"Yes, there are quite a few people going on vision quests in the spring and the fall. On my reservation alone, there were six of them out at one time.

"There are different levels of vision quests. Sometimes you can just go for a walk and meditate so that you can get close to nature. There is a strength in tranquility and peace. They provide energy.

"If one wishes to go on the full vision quest, complete with fasting and the seeking of a guide and a vision, he walks in the footsteps of the saints throughout history who have communicated with God, the Great Spirit. The Biblical figures did it; the Indians do it."

Again, I suppose, some might raise the criticism that modern man should emulate neither the spiritual practices of the prophets of two thousand years ago nor the lifestyle of "untutored savages" of several hundred years ago. How would you answer such a charge?

"One time I gave a lecture in Omaha on the Indian religion. During the question and answer period, an anthropologist asked me, 'How can you say such glowing things about the Native American religion? How can you say that they were not savages? Isn't it true that some tribes practiced human sacrifice?'

"I answered, 'You have to examine the reasons why these tribes offered a human life in sacrifice. I have researched this practice among the Indians in Mexico, and I will admit that there were four tribes in the

United States which practiced human sacrifice. In fact, there was one of them as near to us as Kansas, where they offered a pure person—and it wasn't always a virgin maiden, either. Why did they do this? There were three basic reasons: one, so that they could retain their way of life; two, so that they would have successful crops and prosperity; and three, so that enemy tribes would not war on them.

"Savagery or barbarism is really a relative term when one examines history from its beginnings. How do we retain such elements today in our dominant society? We put thousands of young men in uniform and have them slaughtered, desecrated, so that we can retain our way of life, so that we will maintain economic stability and prosperity, so that enemy nations will not war on us. I ask you, who is really the greater savage?

"The anthropologist sat down very quietly. The rest of the audience was applauding."

That is a very good parallel. Chief Eagle, what is your opinion of the Native American Church?

"It has its rightful place, but I do feel it is misnamed. A Native American church should emphasize traditionalism and traditional principles. I feel there is too much infringement of Christianity in their church. I feel a proper title would be the Native American Christian Church."

What is your opinion of Wovoka, the Peace Messiah, and the Ghost Dance?

"I don't think Wovoka was a trickster. I think he knew himself that he was not a messiah. I think that was a label conjured up by other people. He had a prophetic message for people. I think we should all take another look at what Wovoka was teaching. The press and the federal system corrupted what he was saying, what he was trying to do for the Indian people. Let us look at what he said, rather than at what happened after his words were corrupted."

Sitting Bull and the Sioux are usually given the discredit for that particular corruption. It was said that Sitting Bull was looking for a method of rousing his people to rebellion and seized upon the magic of the Ghost Dance.

"I really can't agree with that theory. I think the Sioux agreed that Wovoka had a real message of peace. Wovoka's dance was supposed to bring down what the Christians would name the 'grace of God.' It was the white press and the white settlers' fear that transformed the ritual into a savage war dance."

Is there a place in the Lakota theology for such a concept as reincarnation?

"Reincarnation is something that not too many Indians talk about."

Do you have a feeling of having been reborn? Do you feel you might have had an earlier life as an American Indian?

"Some of the elders have told me that, although no one knows what Crazy Horse looked like, they feel that if I had been living in those days, I would have been just like Crazy Horse. But they tell me in this life, at least, I have a chance to live a long time!"

I find Crazy Horse one of the most fascinating figures in American history. He was a solitary person who always followed his own medicine. If he had been born a whiteman, he would have been regarded as an eccentric, perhaps a fool. Among the tolerant Sioux, there is provision for someone following his own medicine, so Crazy Horse could become a great leader, a warrior-mystic. I know that even today he is regarded as a great figure among the Indian people.

"He certainly is. You know, although he finally did surrender to the United States government, he never did sign a treaty, because he did not trust the system.

"As soon as he surrendered, he was asked to go with his men up to the north country to help defeat Chief Joseph of the Nez Perce. This saddened Crazy Horse, but he said that he would go. He first gave a speech that is one of the most moving that I have ever heard. It is even more inspiring than Chief Joseph's famous speech. I must properly translate Crazy Horse's speech, because it was a mistranslation of his words that got him killed.

"An interpreter said that, within the speech, Crazy Horse said, 'I will take my warriors to the north country, and I will fight until all the cavalrymen are dead.' Crazy Horse had actually said words to the effect that if the Great Father, the President, willed it, he would take his warriors to the north and fight alongside the cavalrymen, so that the wars might be ended, that all killing would cease, that they might all live in peace.

"When General Crookes, whom the Indians called General Crooked Three Stars, heard the faulty translation, he, or someone on his staff, gave orders to eliminate Crazy Horse."

But it was a red soldier who bayoneted Crazy Horse.

"It was a whiteman, Brad. There were too many witnesses among the Sioux prisoners who could testify to that truth. Crazy Horse died in his father's arms. His father's name was Wound."

Is it true that no one knows where Crazy Horse is buried?

"That is true. Indian mystics have told me that I could find exactly where he is buried. Some people know the area, but they say I can find the exact spot."

Would you ever do this?

"What good would it do? The system would just want to dig him up so that they might examine the remains and find out what he looked like."

Why are the Black Hills considered sacred to the Lakota?

"Because before the Great Invasion, everything the Indians desired could be found in the Black Hills. They believed that the Black Hills was the very heart throb of the Earth Mother. I think my book *Winter Count* tells you the feelings of the Indians about the Black Hills."

What would you say was the essence of the Lakota world view?

"Humanhood. Treating your fellow man as a brother. Indians believe that all men are related and that we are only passing through this life as an exercise in dealing with our fellow man. How one treats his fellow man is a determining factor in how he elevates his inner spirit."

Every student of Native American culture has heard references to the legend of the White Buffalo. Occasionally, novels and motion pictures of frontier life will include scenes depicting the native peoples' "superstitious awe" of the sacred white buffalo. Here, for the first time, Dallas Chief Eagle has translated and shared the actual legend as it was set forth in the oral tradition of the Lakota people. The words are both powerful and beautiful in their simplicity. Do not be blocked from absorbing the universal and timeless relevance of the legend's message by the protective shield of pseudo-sophistication, which more often than not clouds understanding of "primitive myths." This legend has been repeated to countless generations as a teaching device. Do not be afraid to learn from wise ones who have long ago made their journey to the Spirit World.

My relation, I am an old man now, and I have seen many seasons file by like an animal procession to a water pond. Hear my tongue, my brother, for I have chosen this last sunset to tell you of an ancient legend. I feel the dawn will not follow the twilight of my life. When I sleep I will awake in the beyond, where there is no darkness.

This sacred legend had its beginning many winters before the Great Invasion from the dawn country. To ensure its continuation this legend is always handed down by men whose minds and eyes are wise and kind, men acquainted with sacred chants and meditations. This is why its exactness has never vanished. Being the present bearer, I hand down to you the "Legend of the White Buffalo." I hope your mind is ready to bind it for the next generation.

In an age before we had horses, in a season of budding spring, two braves went out scouting for the buffalo. For three days they hunted and tracked over plain, hill, and valley. On the fourth day, following the sunrise, the braves caught sight of a buffalo herd in a valley on the eastern stretch of the mountains. The herd was scattered across the valley.

The two hunters rushed their descent into the valley, and through habit of many hunts, slowed their pace as they neared the buffalo. Then it was, with equal surprise and joy, they noticed the white buffalo in the center of the herd. White with fur like winter etching, the prairie monarch stood motionless, enveloped in mystic vapor.

The hunters paused to robe themselves in wolf and coyote hides to kill their human odor, and readied their weapons. The buffalo throughout the valley began to move toward the White Buffalo, forming a circle around the White One. The two hunters moved cautiously toward an opening on the eastern side of the circle.

The music of nature does not fly in discord, and it was all around the valley. As the hunters crept closer to the opening in the herd, the spirit of the White Buffalo fully enveloped them, causing them to forget their desire to kill.

When the crouching hunters reached the opening, a blinding white flash brought them up straight. In place of the White Buffalo stood a beautiful woman in complete whiteness. In sunlight grandeur, she stood with hands extended, and the soft whisper of the wind made her hair, white skin, white robe, and white buckskin dress shimmer radiantly. Her mouth moved, and her voice, gentle and warm, flowed with a depth of sympathy that brought quiet to the valley.

> I was here before the rains and the violent sea.
> I was here before the snows and the hail.
> I was here before the mountains and the winds.
> I am the spirit of Nature.
>
> I am in the light that fills the earth, and in the darkness of nighttime.
> I give color to nature, for I am in nature's growth and fruits.
> I am again in nature where themes of mystic wisdom are found.
> I am in your chants and laughters.
> I am in the tears that flow from sorrow.
> I am in the bright joyous eyes of the children.

> I am in the substance that gives unity, completeness, and oneness.
> I am in the mountains as a conscious symbol to all mankind when earth's face is being scarred with spiritual undone.
> I am in you when you walk the simple path of the redman.
>
> I am in you when you show love of humankind, for I also give love to those who are loving.
> I am in the response of love among all humans, for this is a path that will find the blessing and fulfillment of the Great Spirit.
>
> I must leave you now to appear in another age, but I leave you with the redman's path.

Complete stillness was everywhere. The White Buffalo Spirit withdrew her hands, and with a glowing smile of eternal love, her body began to return to vapor.

One hunter could no longer contain himself from the beauty of the White Buffalo Spirit. His mind filled with extreme desire. He flung his weapons aside, brushed off his robe, and rushed for the fading spirit. A blinding flash again filled the circle. The White Buffalo Spirit was gone; the White Buffalo was gone; and all that remained was the skull of the charging hunter, gray ashes, and his formless bones.

This, my brother, is why we hold the White Buffalo to be sacred. The White Buffalo moves without the threat of an arrow or lance, whether we sight him in the northern forest, the plains country, or in the mountain regions.

I hope that your tongue can interpret the deep wisdom of this holy legend, and that you, my brother, may help to bring its message to all mankind.

11
Chippewa Medicine Man

The first time Sun Bear, founder of the Bear Tribe Medicine Society, and I met in person, his medicine helper Wabun had to separate us.

The reason for the forceful disentanglement was not due to our inability to strike a harmonious relationship or our inability to communicate effectively with one another. To the contrary, from the moment I had entered his mobile home lodge outside of Reno and had been embraced as a brother, we had not stopped talking. It seemed as though we were compelled to share a lifetime of experiences, visions, and dreams with one another before the sun could rise on a new day.

"Come on, Sun Bear," Wabun attempted to growl around an indulgent smile, "Brad and Dave Graham have traveled nearly two thousand miles to talk with you. They're not going to vanish during the night. Why not get some sleep so you can talk all day tomorrow?"

Sun Bear laughed and placed Igamu, the cat he had been stroking, on the floor.

"You see," he told us, "the woman does not just keep to the background among the Indians. She has always been allowed to voice her opinion concerning any matter. The Indian woman has always had equality. That is why the whiteman fabricated this tale about the terrible slavery of the 'squaw'. He didn't want his own women to find out about women's lib any sooner."

Sun Bear scooped up two sleeping bags from a storage area off the kitchen. "Here, brothers," he smiled, "we will treat you like tribesmen. No fancy beds."

Dave and I answered that we would consider such treatment to be an honor. Sun Bear and Wabun waved their good nights. Richard and

Helen had turned in long ago. Ronnie, a young Chippewa, had taken her bedroll to the Volkswagen bus next to the lodge.

There was a mattress on the floor or a couch against a wall. Since Dave's height is four inches above my own six feet, I volunteered to curl up on the couch. From the inquiring look in Igamu's eye, we knew that the cat would probably take turns sleeping with both of us.

I don't really think I slept at all that night. Sun Bear's soft earnest voice and his recounting of ancient Chippewa prophecies and his own visions were very much with me.

Sun Bear seemed to generate a vortex of power, and the heavy medicine vibrations of the Bear Tribe's encampment had suffused me with a kind of energy that made it very difficult to lie down and turn everything off until the daylight hours. I tried concentrating on the strong wind that sang a power chant of its own, as it rose and dipped in tone and volume, promising snow and cold and urging the completion of any winter preparations. But even listening to the windsong, a sleep-fetching device I had employed with some degree of success ever since I was a boy, failed to lull me into anything more than a state of physical relaxation and a sense of well-being. My body rested, but my brain was actively framing dozens of questions for Sun Bear to answer.

Then time became a blur, and Sun Bear was once again before me, slouched in an old easy chair, legs crossed, a cup of tea cradled in his large, work-worn hands.

"We'll talk off and on between my work," he said. "There is much to do."

I nodded over the rim of my cup. Wabun had told us to come and stay as long as we liked, but that work for the Bear Tribe would have to continue as if there were no guests in the camp. One cannot expect more from busy people.

"We got a lot of walnuts yesterday when we came back from the craft show," Sun Bear said. His boots were still caked with mud, and he seemed to notice my observation of them. He laughed when he told me that the walnut grove had been so muddy that Wabun had come out of her shoes, and he had let her get her stockings good and wet and muddy before he had carried her to dry ground. "Mud can help us connect with the Earth Mother," he said.

"Many people let us pick up what they consider leftovers," Sun Bear explained. "We are not too proud to take them. With the heavy times ahead, at some point everyone will have to learn to become a good forager."

Sun Bear placed a sack of walnuts between his knees and grabbed a paring knife. "I will remove the covering from the walnuts, and you ask me questions."

He squeezed the rotting pulp from the nut, laughed as the dark stain covered his fingers. "Hey, I can rub this juice on me and become as dark as an Indian!"

Do some people come to you and expect to see you walking around in white buckskins with a pious expression on your face?

"Oh, yes, quite often. I think they leave in disappointment because I don't bring out my rattle and shake it for them. They want me to give with some mumbo-jumbo to make me seem more real to them."

Your point is that medicine is all of you.

"Yes."

I asked Sun Bear to tell me about his childhood. He smiled, sat in reflective silence for a few moments, then reached for a fresh sack of walnuts to husk.

"I was born in northern Minnesota, and I was brought up on the White Earth Chippewa Reservation.

"I was about six years old when I got my first sling shot, and maybe I was about seven years old when my brother Howard taught me how to trap weasel. We would set traps in the culverts on the way to school. By the time I was nine years old, I had my first .22 rifle. I learned to appreciate it on the basis of what it was. It was a tool like an ax or a hoe.

"We lived and hunted pretty much off the land, and in a few years I had 16- and 20-gauge shotguns. We had a few head of cattle, and we cut some pulp cord wood to make a living. When I got a bit older, I would make $400 a year trapping muskrats.

"Sometimes when I was about sixteen, I would go out and work on the farms in North Dakota. We worked on pitching bundles. This was during the last of the threshing before the combines came in. Those German and Russian farmers out there in North Dakota are really good workers. We might start at four o'clock in the morning. We would hitch up our teams and haul in bundles for threshing. The old tractor was there, but the horses brought them in. We got about eighty-five cents an hour. It was hard work, but I enjoyed it.

"My dad had sheep and cattle, so we used to put up hay. He also used to cut wood and sell it in the cities. We would work out in the potato fields to make money, too.

"We kids went to a country school south of Lengby, Minnesota. There were both Indian and non-Indian kids there, and it wasn't any heavy trip whether you were Norwegian or not. I learned to appreciate a lot of those Scandinavian dishes. I think all of us kids grew up with respect for each other.

"When I turned seventeen, I started to work in some of the towns around there. I went to Fargo, Grand Forks, other places. I worked in a cemetery, a bakery. I finally got a pretty good job working for a garment company out of Chicago selling factory-direct suits. We would go from one town to another, selling made-to-measure suits. This gave me a way of traveling around, and I enjoyed it.

"In about 1950, a group of us Indian people formed the White Buffalo Council in Fargo. We wanted to have something we could do together and work on together. We would have meetings, powwows, get together to smoke the pipe and talk things out.

"In 1953, I was involved with the Wichita Warriors Club, but prior to that time, I had a thing with the United States Government.

"Many white people are under the impression that Indian people don't have to go into the army, but the reservations were subject to the draft the same as anywhere else. They kept pushing me to go into the army. I was in there about three months when they started talking about this Korean thing. I was willing to get my duty in, but I was not about to fight Koreans. The Koreans hadn't taken anything from me. We Indians don't feel we have any right to murder people in other countries.

"After about three and a half months, I could see there was no way of reasoning with these people, so I split. I was at Camp Chaffee, Missouri. I had picked up some good pointers on how to handle military equipment. But, basically, this just isn't where we're at. Man can't accomplish anything in reality with that sort of equipment. The thing of it was, the federal government was trying to get us to do its thing.

"After I had split, I spent the time visiting other Indian people. I ended up in Reno after I had been at Santa Rosa working at the apple harvest. I lived with the Pimas. I got a crafts center going. This was way back before the war on poverty was ever heard of. We were trying to bring together a group of people and keep them working.

"I would work picking spuds and onions to keep my eating money coming in, then I would take home an extra bag of onions to the people on the reservation. That was the way the old-timers used to do it. They would share and distribute to everyone according to need.

"I was doing the work I believed in when the FBI came around and picked me up for splitting from the United States Army. I was taken down to the state air force base and flown to Fort Oregon for my sentencing. I got a fifty-seven-page court-martial. It took them a whole day to go through the whole trip on me. Officers' wives and other people were packed in the courtroom to see the scene of it. The word was that I was some kind of Indian Robin Hood.

"The army threatened me with all sorts of things. First, they were trying to say that I was guilty of treason. Not only had I deserted the army, but I had used my influence in talking against the military.

"I got a lawyer who was sympathetic to me. He argued that the whole thing was not a question of my guilt, but that I was a man who had come from another society and that I was consistent with my way of life. It was not a question of guilt, he said, but a question of whether justice would be done. He said the United States Government had a long history of aggression against the American Indian and that those acts should be considered at this time.

"I ended up court-martialed, but it turned out to be an indictment against the United States, because I quoted Sitting Bull and Crazy Horse, and other outstanding Indian leaders. The major who was arguing my case got things down to a year; and due to many of my people in Nevada writing letters and petitions, I got out in seven and one-half months on a military probation thing.

"I went back to Nevada to work with my Indians. We had been in the midst of completing homes and we were building workshops for arts and crafts shows. The army finally decided that I was contributing more working with my people than I would have been vegetating in prison. Here is a poem I wrote during my war-protesting days":

TO WAR! TO WAR!

It's the same cry of fifty centuries or more—the cry of rearm to war, to war. Captains shout and bugles blare
While muskets blast and rockets flare.
First it was the Egyptian Pharaohs host, then mighty Sennacherib with an army of which he boasts;
But down tumbled their kingdom, and Babylon rose high over all;
Then the steel-bowed Mede and Persians brought about its fall.
Greece the cradle of Democracy rose to fame,
Then war between Athens and Sparta came. Now Roman warlords brought bloody history on at a pace
For with their legions they sought to establish a super race.
When out of the North rode the barbarian Hordes,
As the Huns and Turks cut the Roman cords.
Now came mighty Charlemagne upon the scene,
And all Europe was conquered to fulfill his dream.

They said peace at last when treaties of West Holpia were signed,
But peace comes not to heart or mind.
Trouble by day and sorrow by night,
When will men learn that swords seldom bring right?
To the West now shifts the historical scene;
Taxation without representation, revolt will fight the scheme.
Then armies are marching, as a great nation is broken in two.
Two different flags waving,
And uniforms are one of grey, the other blue.
Peace for a time again,
Although small wars are waged every day and always it's sorrow with which the people pay.
But Mars God of War looks down on it all
And says, I'll stir them to battle, make the mighty one fall.
Great ones prepare proudly, the small ones in fright.
By the millions they mass; their banners are many fold.
It seems all Hell's broken loose, and death untold,
For mortar, airplanes, fire, and poison gas
Bring death and destruction to every class.
This is a war to end all wars, the politicians now cry.
After this will be peace; men will not kill and die.
We'll league the nations together, keep peace by disarmament.
This role will be better. But scarce had the din of battle died,
And dictator Hitler was marching with Mussolini by his side.
Blood ran in Spain, as Franco overthrew Governmental power.
Maps changed from day to day, as leaders fled their guiding tower.
But the war was fought and won,
And the Dove of Peace saw a new rising sun.
Then in old friends, new enemies are found,
And the post-war plan of peace is declared out of bound.
How will it stop? Where will it end?
Who knows, for these are but plans for mortal men.
For it is war or peace,
As small nations fight to keep their fleece.
War in Cyprus and the Philippines,
War in Viet Nam, Korea, and elsewhere behind the scenes.
But Oh! we have the United Nations now; and man will bring peace through it somehow.
But can selfish man bring peace to this world of unrest,
Or will he have just smaller wars at best?
So while the Devil fiddles the Nation's dance,
Prepare for the battle, let each soldier sharpen his lance.
And it's the same cry that went forth for fifty centuries or more,
The cry of rearm to war, to war!

Can you tell us about your years in Hollywood?

"I spent about seven years in front of the cameras playing cowboys-and-Indians. I worked on the 'Brave Eagle' series for CBS. At least he was a noble savage. I was technical director on that series. I did some parts, mostly walking around in the background carrying my bow and arrow.

" 'Brave Eagle' was backed by Roy Rogers Productions, and I had been hired direct from the producer's office. I worked when the cameras rolled, regardless.

"One time a new assistant director fired me because I was playing checkers when he thought I should be doing some new chores he had just dreamed up. When I came to work the next day, he asked why I had come back, since he had fired me. I told him that things did not work that way. I was a personal friend of Roy Rogers's horse, Trigger, and I worked whenever the cameras did.

"Russ Scott, Roy Rogers's cousin, and I were two extras who worked all the time. The producers had invented this whole Indian chief trip, and they really needed a technical director.

"They had first spent about $75,000 on a pilot film about Cochise. But then the producer's son, who was a boy scout, informed daddy that Cochise was an Apache, who never wore one of those beautiful Sioux headdresses. That shot the pilot down the drain.

"Mike North, who had the brainchild in the first place, decided that they needed a technical director. They decided to dump Cochise, because that had become a public name, anyway, and create their own chief. They decided it was time to find out about teepees.

"I would read over the script, telling them what should be changed to make it more authentic. Then I would go out on the set and look around. There would be a six-foot drum from the Congo. There would be J.C. Penney Indian-print blankets hanging over the teepee flaps. I got rid of most of that.

"Once Brave Eagle, who was played by Keith Larson, was hiding one of his braves because he had stolen some horses from the Blackfeet. I told Paul Andres, the director, that I did not see the scene at all. He asked me what would be the real scene of it.

" 'Brave Eagle,' I said, 'would be having a dance in honor of his brave for his having gotten his tribe some new horses.'

"Andres told me that Brave Eagle was a property-minded Indian.

"I said, 'Yes, he is the property of CBS!'

"Whenever the six writers who did the series would run out of steam, they would call me and say 'Hey, Sun Bear. Why don't you come and have dinner with us?' They would pump me, and I would lay some ideas on them. The next thing I knew, another script would be out.

"Once they used my name for a character, Chief Sun Bear, and the story ended up illustrated in a Dell, 'Brave Eagle' comic book. I used to tease people that I was star of stage, screen, radio, and comic books.

" 'Brave Eagle' was an interesting thing, and I worked for them for about six months straight. Then I dropped out and came back to work for the Indian people. When I got things squared away again, I came back and went into the 'Broken Arrow' television series, which had Michael Ansara playing good old Cochise.

"I got out of series work after this, and I became a free-lance actor. I even got to where I was grabbing Chinese parts away from the Chinese. I played a Tibetan brother in *Marriage-go-Round,* because I looked more a Tibetan type than anyone they could come up with. In *The Ugly American,* I played the Chinese sergeant who rescues Marlon Brando when the mob at the airport is pounding his Cadillac to pieces.

"But the thing I liked best about television and motion pictures was that they gave me free time to do the work with the Indian people that I really wanted to do. During the time that I was acting, I worked with Indian centers, and I helped the women's clubs hustle money so they could buy boxes of groceries for needy families.

"As I traveled around the country and visited the Indian people, I saw that they were beaten down more on the social scale than any other people. They had little sense of their culture, their heritage. In 1953, many of the Indian groups were considered nothing but a cheap labor source for the surrounding farmers and orchard growers.

"The older people had been pushed through the government schools, and they had no sense of identification with their Indian culture. When my dad went to school, he was beaten if he spoke Indian. Those government schools were set up to divorce the Indian from his culture and to reward those who demonstrated by their attitude that they had turned their backs on Indian ways. If an Indian boy would run away from school and get caught, upon his return he would have to run a line of other Indian boys, lashing at him with military belts.

"The whole philosophy of those Indian schools seemed to be: 'Indian, you are not going to make out as well as a whiteman in this world, but we are going to make you over so that you can at least get some menial-task strips of it.'

"I feel that all labor is honest, and I see nothing wrong with working. But when society takes an entire race of people and conditions them to believe that they are fit only for manual labor and menial tasks, there is something very wrong with the system. If I went in cold to an employment agency, they would probably try to find a pick-and-shovel job for me. It makes no difference that I can write, that I can manage a television station."

Why did you choose to live near Reno, Nevada in 1972?

"That was an area where I could live near the city, make a livelihood with crafts and lecturing, and still be close to the wide-open spaces. We lived on the fringe of the city which, at that time, seemed to put us in a position where we could live off the land. Then Reno started growing, and the water supply stayed the same size. We felt that it was time to move on. First we moved to Klamath Falls, Oregon, where we lived for two years, building a home and farm and helping some of the traditional Klamath people, who were struggling to retain some of their land and culture.

"Then the local officials started poisoning the water in the irrigation ditches to kill the algae. The poison also killed the fish and hurt the land. We decided that it was time to move further north. We came to the Spokane, Washington, area; it felt good to us. In my dreams I was shown that this would be an area where there would be water even when other parts of the country went dry.

"We began to look for land and found twenty acres with a good spring, big rocks, and pines. As soon as we saw it we knew that it was the right place for us to settle and grow. Later we found old petroglyphs from the Spokane Tribe on some rocks at the base of the mountain on which we settled. We found that the old ones called the mountain 'Vision Mountain,' and that it was a traditional place for native people to go for their vision quests. Since we originally moved here, a lot of the surrounding land has been purchased by people who share our direction, who love and respect this sacred mountain as much as we do.

"You know, according to all the ancient Indian prophecies, we see us fast approaching the time of the Great Purification, so it will be important to be able to live off the land. This system is about to come crashing down.

"When we traditional Indian people speak of the end of the whiteman, we are not speaking of a race, we are speaking of a way of life. A dog-eat-dog philosophy.

"You know that my medicine is for brothers and sisters of all races. Throughout the European's involvement with this land and its native peoples, many non-Indians have come to various tribes and have joined them. Even some of the early Jesuit fathers took off their robes and joined the Indians. They said, 'Hey, these people have never read the Book, yet they have it going for them already.'

"I can sympathize and understand the work and medicine and goals of a lot of the militant people, but their great feelings of hostility have grown to the point where they have no trust at all of any non-Indians. I cannot be a part of this, because I feel that we are moving toward a new society, a new way of life. If I were to copy this negative scene and perpetuate the idea of hatred toward another person on the basis of race, I would be imitating the thing I hate most—a rotten system of judgment that has been used to destroy people all over the world.

"The black people in the cities have suffered from this and all the other poison that bigoted stupidity has put down on them. Now the turning point has come. They are going to declare a full vendetta on the system. If this happens, you won't be able to hold up your hand and say 'I am your brother' because all that angry man will see is your face.

"The people who really want to survive the destruction of the system and the Great Purification and who really want to live to find real brotherhood on the Earth Mother again will move away from these situations. That is part of the traditional Indian's warning: *Get away from the cities! Get out where there is safety!*

"It is not a question of whether or not the Great Purification will be. It will. The whole of major cities will be destroyed. If one part of the prophecies is true, then all of the prophecies are true. The major confrontations in the Middle East are part of the plan. The Earth Mother is about to declare her complete rebellion.

"The real thing of brothers and sisters coming together is to get to know one another and to get rid of all those old fears and phobias. That is what we have found.

"Medicine is a part of me, and it does not have to be put off in a separate box. I tell people of the Bear Tribe how we raise crops, dry fruit, put up our stores. Some say, 'We are more interested in learning medicine. We want to go up on the mountaintop.' All others want to know is where the peyote buds are kept.

"First, you have to show respect for the Earth Mother. The making of love, the showing of love for the plants and fruits—these things are all part of medicine. You don't separate medicine from living. That is why the majority of the people in the system, the society that came to this country from across the Great Waters, have never had a religion that has been real to them. They do not take their religion beyond the church building. They never really taste their religion.

"When I make a prayer, when I make medicine, I do not do it only at a certain time. I do it when it is needed. Too many white people in the system are always bugging the Lord to give them something, and all too often they forget to give thanks for the many things they already have.

"I have been to the meetings in churches, and I have heard them praying for television sets, for refrigerators, for new cars. I can see their picture: God is sitting up there answering all these telephone lines, sending out all the goodies. The way I have the picture, he is bursting with laughter and shaking his head.

"Sometimes it is hard to be patient with those who say they want to go to the mountaintop when it is easy to see that they have not worked out a balance here because they are caught up in their own frustrations. Sometimes I tell them, 'How can you go to the mountaintop when you can't solve your emotional problems? You are walking around with a hard-on and you haven't got to where you can relate to other human beings.'

"It is hard to have a relationship with God if you can't function on the level where you recognize that you are each others' brothers and sisters.

"Those who seek a higher understanding of things must first lay a solid foundation and establish a good balance. On the basis of my experience and the experiences of my people, when you go up to make medicine and fast to seek a vision, you are on the level of the Spirit World. If you are held back by all the worries of paying the rent and getting a new car, your mind just won't reach out."

Do you ever feel that you have done all this before?

"Sometimes I have a sense of continuity. Sometimes I will be sitting down, and I see a lot of people that I have seen before. Lots of times I see them on the street. Many brothers, like Dave Graham here, I feel I have seen before."

Does such a concept as reincarnation fit in with medicine power?

"I don't necessarily see this in the words of reincarnation. Too often reincarnation becomes an ego thing.

"I see myself and other people as continuing forces in different forms.

"Then there is the fact that we are all part of a whole. We traditional people are striving to bring this concept out—this sense of being part of a whole and sharing together a sense of responsibility on that basis. We are trying to reach out and put our hands on the shoulders of our brothers and sisters and say that we are all part of the same circle."

12
The Bear Tribe

Sun Bear founded the Bear Tribe as a modern day medicine society of teachers who strive in all aspects of their busy and varied lives to relearn their proper relationship with the Earth Mother, the Great Spirit, and all of their relations in the mineral, plant, animal, and human kingdoms. Tribal members try to share with others those lessons of harmony that they have learned. They also attempt to teach people about the traditional Native American philosophy and prophecies as they relate to contemporary life.

Sun Bear gathered the Bear Tribe in response to his first major vision, which showed him the times of earth changes that lay ahead. His vision corresponded to the ancient prophecies of many of the American Indians people. These prophecies foretold a time when the earth and the forces protecting the earth would turn against those people who had been misusing her—poisoning her soil, her water, and her air with no thought of the generations that would come later. They also told of a time when some members of the dominant society would recognize the folly of their lifestyle and would come to the Native people to learn a better way of life.

"In our prophecies," said Sun Bear, "we were told that our people would lie as if we were dead in the dust for a hundred years or more, and then we would rise up and walk on our hind legs again, teaching others as the rightful keepers and protectors of this land. The time of our teaching has already begun."

Sun Bear began the Bear Tribe in California in the late 1960s. He was teaching at the University of California at Davis, and his medicine told him that it was time to share with people of all races the vision that he had had many years before. Prior to that time he had been told to share his medicine only with other Native people.

"It was hard for me to begin that sharing, but I had to honor my medicine. A lot of people, both Native and white, objected to my sharing with non-Natives. Some still do. I felt like I was standing alone at that time. My vision told me we all had to come together as brothers and sisters, no matter what color skin we have been given," Sun Bear explained.

He began to talk about his vision, and many of the young seekers of the sixties enthusiastically responded. Soon he had over two hundred people living in seventeen donated land bases.

Sun Bear: "The people in the tribe had been together for about six months when my medicine told me to carry the message even further. We were getting lots of publicity and lots of letters.

"I set off cross country to tell people about the times of cleansing, to tell them that people must come together and form groups and become self-reliant. I told them that people must go out on the land, but they must not come to the Earth Mother to perpetuate the same sicknesses, the same selfishness, that they had in the system. They must learn to come there with good hearts and with a real sense of love and respect for each other. I had seen these things. It was my vision to tell people about them.

"When I began the tribe I didn't want to have a lot of rules, because it wasn't the traditional way for there to be a policeman on every street corner. People carried the law within their hearts and disciplined themselves to honor those laws.

"Because of the harm I had seen drunkenness bring to Native people, I asked the tribe to abstain from the use of alcohol. Because of the harm I had seen psychedelics do to the young non-Natives who abused them, I asked people to abstain from those drugs.

"When people take their oath to the tribe, they promise to try to build a true, honest, and loving relationship between each other and the Earth Mother. They also promise to refrain from violence and from destructive possessiveness. I hope that some day we won't have to have any rules or restrictions in the tribe, and that people will learn to govern themselves from within so that nobody has to put outside rules on them. But most people coming from the dominant society have not yet grown to that point.

"I trusted the people I left in California to continue with the work that we had begun, both spiritually and physically. We had good gardens, and we had harvested and dried about four tons of fruits and vegetables that year, largely crops that would otherwise have been wasted. People were trying to learn ceremonies to honor the earth and they were trying to learn a better way of living together. Unfortunately, in my absence some of the brothers had been pressured to go back on a psychedelic drug trip.

"When I came back to the tribe in 1971 after taking that cross-country talking trip, I was heartsick. I couldn't eat. I felt that those I had trusted had betrayed my medicine. Finally, I went up on top of a mountain. I took off all my clothes, because your body is one of the few things that is yours to give. The first thing I saw was an eagle circling around above me. Little clouds were scattered in the sky. A big cloud began moving over. I watched it. A little cloud came out from the big one. It was a very still day, but this cloud came out and began to spin like a whirlwind. After a while, just a little bit of the cloud went back to the big cloud. I had been told what would happen to the Bear Tribe.

"I went back to the camp, and I said that those people who see and want to walk the same path as I do could come with me to Reno to begin a new camp. In Reno there would only be the Bear Tribe and our own medicine. Those who wanted a psychedelic, or some other, trip were not welcome to be with us. We wanted only those who wanted to learn a sense of work, love, and responsibility.

"Only a few people chose to come with me at that time. Some of the others attempted to continue with some of the bases in California, but they did not last long. Others went on to other types of seekings. Over the years we have kept in contact with some of the original Bear Tribers, and we have worked together where we can.

"Soon after the move to Reno, Wabun came from the East Coast to join us. She was really surprised at coming to such a small group, but she hung in there and helped me to redevelop the tribe. I had put all of my personal savings and property into the first year and a half of the tribe, so we had to begin to generate some income.

"We spent the summer of 1972 going to Indian powwows where we sold our books and craft items. We began to write *Many Smokes* again. (While I had been working with the tribe in California, we had ceased publication. Otherwise, *Many Smokes* has been in continuous existence for over twenty years.) Other people came to join us, and Nimimosha, who has worked with me for over sixteen years, stayed in there through all of the changes.

"I had to spend a lot of time contemplating what went wrong with the original tribe, and figure out how we could make it work better. I realized that I had been very innocent in reaching out and accepting anyone who said they wanted to be part of a medicine society. In the old days it wasn't that easy for people to become part of a medicine society. They had to prove that their intention was real by giving their time, energy, and efforts to the society. I realized that today it was even harder for people to make a commitment to anything bigger than themselves, because we all grow up in a society that teaches us to compete for things and to ignore our hearts. I realized that people needed time to grow before they could become a permanent part of the tribe. Today people come to us to visit, and they might have to spend a year, or more, working with us before we decide that it feels good to have them as a member of the tribe.

"Originally, I just supported the tribe. Now we ask people who want to be with us to help with that support. We found that those who gave least often were the ones with the loudest criticisms. Much of the tribal finances come from lectures, craft and book sales, and mail order sales of books. Having these sources of income means that people don't have to go out and work for someone else.

"Before we add an activity to our life we measure how it will affect us and the earth. For instance, we began selling books by mail because, going to powwows, we realized how hard it was for people to find books about Native subjects. There was a need, and we felt that we could help to fill it. We are beginning several cottage industries that will help to support the tribe as it continues to grow.

"We stayed in Reno for about two years, and then moved to Klamath Falls, Oregon. After two years there we felt that it was time to move on. We moved to our place near Spokane, Washington, and we built a house, a barn, a granary, two cabins, a root cellar, a greenhouse, and housing for our animals. We have been here for almost six years now, and it feels like a good place to be. The mountain we are on is a very sacred place. It has a lot of medicine that helps people to come in true contact with the energy of the earth. A lot of people have come to us to go out on their vision quests, and most of them have had very good and powerful experiences.

"We slowly began to add people to the tribe, and now we have nine adults and one little girl who are full members of the tribe. Usually, we also have between five and ten other people living, working, and sharing with us—some of them wanting to become part of the tribe, and some wanting to learn so they can go to other parts of this earth and share with others. About two hundred people come to visit with us on our home base every year.

"After our move to Washington, we began to get a lot of invitations to speak at centers and conferences all over, and we have been doing that. I could be on the road all year if I wanted to be. I probably speak directly to about 20,000 people a year at this point. We also began to give seminars on self-reliance, earth awareness, and the vision quest at our home base, which is near Ford, Washington, about thirty-five miles outside of Spokane.

"The message of my first vision is still the same. The medicine that we see is people coming together as groups and becoming big families or tribes, living together in harmony. We have realized that people have to learn what it is to be a tribe, and that the best way of teaching that is through example.

"People have to learn what it means to have loyalty, love, and sharing with other human beings. They have to learn how good it can feel to open your heart to other two-leggeds, to serve your brothers and sisters, to learn what it means to think of your actions in terms of how they will affect those around you.

"When Native people went out to pray for a vision they always prayed to know how they could best serve their people and the earth. People have to learn this again today, and they have to clean out of their heads all the little selfish trips that keep people feeling separated and afraid of each other. The worst thing about the system is that it separates people. We have been pitted against each other for survival for too long.

"In the Bear Tribe, everyone must work. Medicine has to start with the raising of corn and plants. If your medicine doesn't work there and you don't have things to feed your people regularly, then you really don't have any medicine at all. I often tell people, 'If it doesn't grow corn, I don't want to hear about it.'

"At this point, the tribe is about 60 percent self-sufficient in terms of food production. This year we plan to be even more self-sufficient. We don't yet have enough of the right land to grow our own grains and hay. We raise big gardens, and preserve the food from them. We have planted fruit trees, and we raise cows, chickens, rabbits, pigs, ducks, geese, and goats for meat and dairy products. We see our gardens and animals as part of our medicine. Indian religion was never a segregated kind of thing. It is a way of life. The reality is that everything is one continuous stream of medicine.

"Ultimately we see the time when humanity will walk on the Earth Mother as one big family. There will be respect for one another, and for all of the other beings who live on the earth with us.

"Back in 1977, I was blessed with another vision, one that has helped me to give people more sense of how they fit into this continuous stream of medicine. This was a vision of the return of the ancient Medicine Wheels of the Native people here as well as in other parts of the world.

"In my vision I saw a hilltop bare of trees, and there was a soft breeze blowing. The prairie grass was moving gently. Then I saw a circle of rocks that came out like the spokes of a wheel. Inside was another circle of rocks, nearer to the center of the wheel. I knew that here was the sacred circle, the sacred hoop of my people, the Medicine Wheel. Inside of the center circle was the buffalo skull, and coming up through ravines, from the four directions, were what looked like animals. As they came closer, I saw that they were people wearing headdresses and animal costumes. They moved to the wheel and each group entered it sunwise, making a complete circle before they settled on their place in the wheel.

"All the people were singing the song of their season, of their minerals, of their plants, and of their totem animals. And they were singing songs for the healing of the Earth Mother. A leader among them was saying, 'Let the medicine of the sacred circle prevail. Let many people across the land come to the circle and make prayers for the healing of the Earth Mother. Let the circles of the Medicine Wheel come back.'

"In this vision were gathered people of all the clans, of all the directions, of all the totems; and in their hearts they carried peace. That was the vision I saw.

"Since that vision, we have spread the message of the Medicine Wheels in many ways. My medicine told me that soon after the vision happened we would publish a book explaining the vision and the meaning of the Medicine Wheels. We first printed a circle about the wheels, and Wabun sent a copy of it to her former agent, who was then an editor with Prentice Hall. It arrived on his birthday and he was very taken with it. Soon he asked us if we would write a book. We did, and it was published in 1980.

"That same year we organized and sponsored our first Medicine Wheel gathering near Seattle, Washington. Over six hundred people came together there to join in the ceremony of building a Medicine Wheel. It was a very moving event for me, and for many of the other people there.

"In 1981, we had three large Medicine Wheel gatherings, and we built Medicine Wheels in many parts of this country and in Europe. And many of the people who come to these gatherings go out and build wheels in other places. So it spreads.

"You see, Medicine Wheels are one way of honoring the energy of the earth, of celebrating and strengthening this energy. The old ones knew that you had to give back to the earth, not just take things from her. Medicine Wheels were one such way of giving. I am very thankful for the vision I was given, and for the opportunity to see it grow and help the earth during this time of cleansing."

Nimimosha ("Woman with a Heart of Love"), you have been with the Bear Tribe for sixteen years. How did your association with Sun Bear begin?

Nimimosha: "I met Sun Bear in Berkeley, during the days of the free speech movement. Some friends introduced us, and, after hearing about the work he was doing, and wanted to do, I decided that I wanted to help him. I left Berkeley and moved to Los Angeles to help him with *Many Smokes* magazine, and his other projects.

Why have you stayed with the tribe?

"Working with the tribe gives me a real feeling of accomplishment, both on a personal level and on a larger level. Being with the tribe has helped me to develop my view of the world. My prior background was very much white, middle-class. When I saw that there was more to the world than that, I wanted to participate in it. I feel that my involvement with the tribe is a constructive way to be part of meaningful things that are happening."

What is it that Sun Bear is doing that makes you feel that there is more here than working with some other group?

"I am loyal to the tribe, but the tribe is also loyal to me. We watch out for each other, support each other in growing. Such a sense of loyalty is rare in a society where everyone is so competitive."

How would you articulate the ideals of the tribe?

"We feel a sense of responsibility to each other and to the earth. We also have a responsibility to teach others about the earth, and the times of cleansing. And we have a personal responsibility to grow and to develop our individual potentials."

What was the biggest adjustment that you had to make?

"None of the adjustments were bad because they came gradually. When I first met Sun Bear, the tribe didn't exist. This was something we built together, with some of the other good people who came to join us later."

Sun Bear: "Many people at that time were coming to me and wanting to join me, but I didn't really have anything for them to come and join. I didn't feel the need at that time to go through with what we are doing now. At that time, I tried to help people by telling them about living in harmony with their brothers and sisters on the Earth Mother. A good relationship between brothers and sisters is so important, because if you can't accomplish this, you can't begin to reach higher."

Nimimosha: "The system in which I grew up had alienated me. It offers such a competitive trip that some people are left in the dust with no assurance that they are going to survive. The Bear Tribe is a group that is interested in survival, but we are not interested in enriching ourselves at our brothers' and sisters' expense.

"For instance, someone just asked if she could use my sewing machine. Well, it is not really my sewing machine. It is a piece of equipment that belongs to the tribe that happens to be in my custody. We've found that we do not need to be selfish and competitive. There is no need for it. I think we are going to be working on this shared feeling even more. Sharing works; caring works; and the competitive system doesn't."

What about the spiritual aspects of the tribe. Are they meaningful to you?

"Of course. We have circles each day, before meals and in the evenings. We smudge [purify with the smoke from burning herbs] each morning. We have our sweat lodge ceremonies every week; and, we have ceremonies to celebrate the changing of the seasons, the elements, the planting of our gardens, and the harvesting of our crops. We try to remember that everything we do is spiritual. And many of us in the tribe have our own private spiritual practices which add another dimension to our daily lives. To be able to breathe real air and go out and see the earth and mountains makes me happier and certainly elevates me spiritually."

Do you find it possible to carry your medicine back into the city?

"Sometimes I find it difficult to practice anything surrounded by dirt, noise, clutter, and insanity. I grew up on a farm in Rhode Island; so, it is hard for me to adjust to a city and to be happy there. I try, though, because I know that the medicine can work any place that you allow it to."

What about those who might accuse you of being a hopeless romantic and suggest that since you couldn't make it in contemporary society, in the city where the action is, you are desperately clutching to some dream life?

"If you are interested in surviving in the system, then what we have out here would be a dream. But we are more interested in teaching people that there is a viable alternative to the system, a way of life with more honor and respect for all of the beings around you. In Sun Bear and the Bear Tribe, I believe there is something more realistic, more lasting than the system."

[Wabun ("East Wind, Woman of the Dawn"), Sun Bear's medicine helper, was born Marlise James thirty-six years ago in Newark, New Jersey. She is a graduate of the Columbia University Graduate School of Journalism, the author of *The People's Lawyers,* and co-author of *The Bear Tribe's Self-Reliance Book,* and *The Medicine Wheel.*]

"I have been writing since I was seven, professionally since I was fifteen. I worked as editor and managing editor of several new-youth magazines that went under during the recession. I started writing *The People's Lawyers* because I was interested in becoming a lawyer myself. I had been a politically active person involved in the peace movement and the woman's movement.

"I was at the point in my life where I was searching for a spiritual direction. I went out to California to talk to some lawyers I was featuring in my book, and there I heard about the Bear Tribe. I didn't have time to follow through, but I kept in touch with a friend who was following the activities of the tribe. I heard from him that Sun Bear was coming east, and I decided to see if I could interview him for a magazine article.

"When I met Sun Bear I knew he was offering the spiritual path I was seeking. I finished my book, and, five months later, came out to Reno to join the tribe. I knew something had happened in California but I didn't realize the extent of the changes brought about in the tribe until I got there. I was expecting to come to a group of two hundred, and found, instead, a group of twelve or so. Nonetheless, I decided to stay and do what I could to help the tribe grow again, in as positive a way as possible."

Was it difficult to make the transition from a New York writer to a member of the tribe?

"You bet. I was a real city girl. The second day I was out west I helped to skin some rabbits, and I was afraid I'd get sick; but, I learned. When I began to help with the garden that first year, I started to feel at home.

Putting my hands into the earth seemed a very natural and healing thing. When I got over being terrified of the insects, snakes, and other things that were strange to me, I began to feel good being out on the earth. I even came to accept the 'strange' things as my relations, my brothers and sisters. When I could do that, my view of the world expanded greatly."

What is there about Sun Bear that really makes all this retribalization work?

"You rarely meet people who truly have a direction in life. Most of us are flopping around all over the place. Most people are looking for a direction, but they don't know how to find it, and, if they do, they are afraid to commit themselves to it. Sun Bear is a man with a vision, and he is truly committed to it. That sets him apart in this world."

What do you think would be the hardest adjustment for someone to make who comes from the system into the tribal structure?

"It seems to be hard for people to learn to take responsibility for their own lives. We've grown up learning to take orders from someone. In the tribe we tell people that they have their own relationship with the Great Spirit and their own responsibility for how they carry that relationship out on the earth. We don't tell them what their vision should be. We ask them to go out and seek it themselves. We tell them what work needs to be done; but we don't stand there and watch them do it. It's hard for some people to accept that much responsibility.

"From my years of experience in watching people come to the tribe it seems that they also have difficulty learning to eliminate competitiveness, learning to take true responsibility, and learning to open their heart to others—to take off their masks and let people see what is underneath. In the tribal ideal, competitiveness, irresponsibility, and hiding are not necessary. Each person is free to be himself or herself as long as he or she measures how his or her actions effect the tribe, the earth, and the generations to come."

Wabun, you are now Sun Bear's medicine helper, director of the tribal businesses, and a well-known lecturer on earth and female energy. How did this all come about in your life with the tribe?

"It all unfolded in a very natural way. I have always been a very high energy person, and one of the things I appreciate about Sun Bear and the tribe is that I've always been given the space to use my energy in the most creative ways I could imagine.

"I began to help Sun Bear with ceremonies very soon after I joined the tribe and was given my name. This responsibility grew as my ability to handle it grew. Helping with ceremonies soon seemed a very natural thing for me to do. I now have the responsibility of directing the ceremonies at the Medicine Wheel gatherings, and it is a real honor to be able to do so—to be able to share with others the sense of how ceremonies can help the earth, and how they can help people feel their sense of oneness with the universe.

"Medicine helpers are also called servants of the medicine, and being in this position has helped me to feel the privilege that it is to be able to serve the earth and your brothers and sisters.

"In the time I've been with the tribe I have, at one time, done just about every job there is to do here—from farm work, to office work, to house work, to communicating with and counselling people. I've enjoyed doing all of them, and I have learned a tremendous amount from doing them. At this time I am working with the tribal businesses because they need a bit more organization, and I have a mind capable of organizing. Last year I spent a good deal of time working on setting up the Medicine Wheel gatherings. The year before I did a lot of writing. Now we have people working with us on the gatherings, so I am able to give that away and move on to working in the business area. When that is organized, and there are more people working with them, I will be working to expand Bear Tribe Publishing. Now we publish three books—*The Self-Reliance Book,* Sun Bear's *Buffalo Hearts,* and *Snowy Earth Comes Gliding,* by Evelyn Eaton, who is a Metis pipe woman, and our tribal grandmother.

"For the past five years I have also been spending a lot of time lecturing with Sun Bear. As I talked to people I found that a lot of what I had to share was about earth and female energy. A lot of people are afraid of these energies today, and they have to realize that their fears are part of the reason for the cleansing of the earth.

"I had a background in the woman's movement, but what I talk about now is very different from the political themes I knew about before. I tell people how female energy reflects the energy of the earth, and how it must be balanced within each individual, no matter what gender we wear. Personal balancing of our energies is a very important part of preparing for the cleansing, and of growing and evolving in life.

"I'm very grateful to the tribe for the personal growth and development it has brought to my life. I feel what we are building in our own community and communicating to others is a positive way of relating to the world around us. It's a challenging life, but a very worthwhile one."

[Shawnodese ("South Wind") is also Sun Bear's medicine helper. Born Thomas More Huber, he graduated from the University of California at Berkeley, and did graduate work at Humboldt State University in Arcata, California. He is a musician and craftsperson who has worked in writing, computer technology, and environmental health. He has also taught yoga, meditation, and guided visualizations.]

Shawnodese, how did you come to be with the Bear Tribe?

Shawnodese: "I had a spontaneous vision about ten years ago, promising many things, including a dramatic life change in my thirtieth year. When I was twenty-nine I was working as a health inspector in Boise, Idaho. I was board president of the Church of Religious Science, active in Unity, and on the board of Inner Forum, a group sponsoring workshops and seminars on spiritual topics. In my spare time I was giving psychic readings and teaching astrology, numerology, meditation, and yoga.

"I was on vacation from the Health Department and teaching a sunrise yoga class on a beach in Hawaii for a Unity retreat. During a relaxation period on the third day, I suddenly realized that the life I was living in Boise would never bring me to the path I had been shown in my first vision. I had the feeling that, if I uncomplicated my life and cleaned up my body through fasting, I would somehow be able to get back in touch with my vision. I began planning the necessary steps as I saw them, and I thought I might come back to Hawaii for the fasting period.

"Back in Boise I began actively moving towards my goal. Then one month later, I met Sun Bear and Wabun for the second time at a seminar. Sun Bear talked to me and invited me to come to the tribe and go out on a vision quest as a Native person would, seeking clarification of my original vision. I finished up my business in Boise and came to the tribe.

"I had a head full of possible plans for fulfilling my life direction and, at that time, I had no thoughts of staying with the tribe. I lived with the tribe for a short time before going out on my quest and felt very at-home there—here were people living together as I thought people should.

"As the day approached for me to begin my vision quest I had tentatively added 'staying with the Bear Tribe' as one of my possible alternatives.

"Then Sun Bear placed me out on the mountain, and I went for four days and nights without food or water, crying for a vision. In both dreams and in a vision, I saw myself living and working with the tribe. When I came back I waited four more days before talking about my experience. The dreams continued, and at last I surrendered. I asked Sun Bear and the tribe if I could stay with them, and they told me the Council of Elders had already met and voted to accept me. I was back on my path once again."

How long ago was that? What has your life been like since that time?

"I went on the vision quest in the summer of 1979. Since I've been with the tribe I've had many responsibilities. I've worked on the farm, learned to care for farm animals, had the opportunity to put theories I knew about farming into practice. I've also done bookkeeping for the tribe, helped with the businesses, and worked on many writing projects. During the last two years I have travelled with Sun Bear and Wabun, lecturing, doing individual counselling, and keeping track of the finances.

"At the tribe I have been able to use a lot of the knowledge that I brought with me—from doing counselling and guided meditations, to helping the tribe learn how to set yearly goals. I am now the sub-chief of the tribe in charge of helping the community and all of the individuals in it to grow in all the ways they can—spiritually, emotionally, mentally, and physically. I am also working with Sun Bear on developing his apprentice program, which is a way for people in all areas and walks of life to share in some of the knowledge that we have."

[The Bear Tribe can be contacted at P.O. Box 9167, Spokane, WA 99209. They ask you to enclose a stamped, self-addressed envelope.]

Can you tell us something about the best ways to store food and other necessities for survival during the coming times of crisis?

Sun Bear: "It is our belief that only those people living on the land in groups in harmony with each other and the Earth Mother will survive the coming cleansing of the Earth. And for these groups to survive, they must be prepared. That means that they must have stored enough supplies to sustain the group for a period of three or more years.

"What will you need to survive? First of all, water. If you have chosen your land well, you will have a good natural water supply that will flow without interruption. A spring or well is the best alternative. If you get your water from a stream it might be cut off or become unsafe during certain periods of the cleansing of the Earth. To make sure you'll have some water if such periods arise you should fill some glass or plastic containers with fresh water, store in a safe place, and check every few months for leaks and freshness. Figure on a minimum of one-half gallon of water per person per day for drinking. To use water that is unsafe, purify it by boiling for one to three minutes, then pour it from one container to another several times to get some air and flavor back in. You may also purify it by adding any bleach that has hypochlorite as its only active ingredient (eight drops to a gallon of clear water, sixteen if the water is cloudy) letting the water sit for a half hour and checking that the chlorine smell is still there. If it isn't, add another dose of the bleach and let stand for another fifteen minutes. You may also use 3 percent tincture of iodine. Add twelve drops to a gallon of clear water, and twice that to cloudy. Or you can use water purification tablets if you have them.

"If you live in the city, you should also be sure to have at least a five-gallon container of water in storage, and you should rotate it at least monthly.

"You should have on hand any herbs or prescription medicine needed by members of your group. If you are able to obtain any strong antibiotics, these might also be helpful. Where possible have a good medical kit, both herbal and allopathic, on hand. Then, of course, you'll need food, seeds, canning and drying equipment, fishing and hunting gear. Having a varied diet is very essential to keeping your balance, so we really urge any of you who think you can live completely off the land to rethink your plan. While you can get your meat through hunting, and forage for wild greens, berries, herbs, and fruits, we believe that more variety than that is necessary. If you have a good supply of seeds, you can grow your own vegetables, then can or dry them for the fall, winter, and spring when you can't get them fresh. Besides canning equipment (remember to have three or four times the number of lids as jars and rings) you'll need sugar or honey for canning fruits and jams, and vinegar, dill, and spices for pickling.

"Because growing a garden may be difficult or impossible for a year or two we suggest that you have canned foods, and dried ones, on hand. For a family of five you'll need, on the average, two cans of soup per day, two of vegetables, one meat, and two fruit, plus five cans of juice per week. In addition, for a year you'll need at least twelve three-pound cans of shortening, six cans of baking powder, and four gallons of Clorox for water purification. (We also suggest that you store a good supply of alfalfa and other seeds for sprouting, and spirulina, a rich source of vegetable protein.)

"Besides your fruits, juices, and vegetables you'll also need some staples. With a mixed diet an adult will use three hundred pounds of wheat per year, or one hundred pounds of flour. Wheat is cheaper to get and easier to store than flour. Make sure to get a hand-powered grinder with a stone burr to grind the wheat. Each adult will also need eighty pounds of powdered milk, one hundred fifty pounds of dried beans and peas (including soybeans, your best nonmeat source of protein), sixty pounds of sugar, fifty pounds of honey, and fifty pounds of peanut butter per year. In addition to the above, store any items that you're used to having in your diet: for instance, coffee, tea, herbs for tea, oats, rice, barley, nuts, hard candies, salt, pepper, spices, vinegar, oil, dessert mixes, corn meal, potatoes, syrup, molasses. To figure out how much you need to store, mark boxes or jars and see how much you use over a two-week period and figure that amount times twenty-six for a year's supply. Store things that will keep well and store them in moisture-, mouse-, and insect-proof containers wherever possible.

"What hunting and fishing gear you'll need depends on what you are used to and can use. A .22 is a good all-around gun, but you have to be a good shot to get small game with it. Shotguns are good for that. Get the right ammunition for the guns you have and get plenty of it. For fishing get plenty of line, an assortment of hooks, flies, sinkers, and a float. You can make your own pole, and, later, your own flies. In case you hit a period where no game is available to you, we suggest having a supply of jerky, dried fish, and canned meat and fish on hand.

"You should also have in storage (or in use) tools that you are likely to need. These should include a good case skinning knife, a sharpening stone, a double-bit ax, a saw, shovel, hammer, screwdrivers, nails, screws, hoe, spade, pliers, pots, pans, plates, bowls, silverware, long-handled fork, matches, several canvas tarps or large pieces of heavy plastic, a fire grill, canteens, rope, washboard, pails. And you should stock up on sanitary and personal items: soaps of all kinds, disinfectants, cleaning solutions, toilet paper, sufficient bedding for everyone, personal clothes, sweaters, heavy jackets, and rain ponchos, sewing equipment, craft supplies, good hiking or woodsman boots, boots or overshoes for winter, work gloves, tooth equipment (include dental floss), sanitary napkins or tampons, towels, extra underwear, alcohol, ammonia, aspirin, bandages, Band-Aids, cotton, ear drops, epsom salts, paregoric, safety pins, shampoo, thermometers, tweezers, antihistamine, liniment, calamine lotion, Vaseline, snake-bite kits, insect repellent, and vitamins. You'll probably also want reading and writing material, cards and other games.

"You'll also need to store different fuels to combat the present fuel shortages, and the worse ones that we'll face in the future. Gasoline is a good fuel that can power not only your car but generators and various other things as well. It can be stored in the metal gasoline cans made specifically for that purpose, or in metal drums. For reasons of both safety and security it is probably best to bury the drums, and not let people see what you are doing. Unleaded gasoline can also be used to fuel Coleman stoves and lanterns. We don't feel that either natural or propane gas will be available for use for much longer, nor do we recommend storing them. Other than gasoline, the only other fuel we feel will be relevant is wood (or possibly coal if you're in an area where it is available). Wood is a good fuel for both heating and cooking, and it is easily available in most areas. We think that you'll be safe if you just have a year's supply ready in advance. In any case, you should always get in your winter's supply before it gets too wet and cold to do so. Four to eight cords of wood should be enough for the heating and cooking needs of a four-room cabin, depending on the area in which the cabin is located. For additional light needs you should have a good supply of candles, flashlights, batteries, kerosene lanterns, and, of course, kerosene.

"We know that we've suggested storing a substantial amount of goods of all kinds and that it will be costly to do so. However, we can't think of any safer investment you can make. While we are geared to having small groups together on the land, we feel that you should start storing these supplies wherever you are and whatever your family structure. But we do urge city dwellers to at least think of places in the country where they might be able to store some of their supplies. We think you should start gathering your storage supplies now. While we can't put a date on when we think the system will destroy itself completely, we don't think there is much time left. And it's better to have your survival supplies ready a year too early rather than an hour too late."

13
Practicing Medicine Power

Let us visualize the following scene: It is a pleasant autumn night. The leaves have turned from green to brilliant daubs of red and gold. The moon is full, and only a few clouds occasionally screen its light. The air is chill enough to make one appreciate a warm jacket or sweater and to encourage one to move closer to the campfire. Twylah has just poured herself another cup of coffee, and she holds the steaming pot over your own cup. Sun Bear is filling his pipe with *kinnikinick*, the native tobacco made of herbs. Dallas Chief Eagle is reaching for a fresh cigarette. The talk is about to turn to that of how one might best practice medicine power.

Sun Bear: "Medicine power to our people means many things. Medicine is different herbs to be used in healing. There is the sweat lodge. There are various healing poultices. It is when the medicine man has the particular gift of knowledge that enables him to go into the medicine lodge and talk to the spirits. All these things are medicine.

"My own thing is that I smoke a pipe and ask for medicine. Sometimes I smoke it all the way through and ask for medicine. Sometimes when energy forces are being used against me, I will smoke my pipe and hold them back."

Would you explain the medicine coins you carry?

Sun Bear: "My medicine coins were given to me as a gift by a bronco Apache. The bronco Apaches are brothers who travel back and forth across the line from Mexico and the United States. They have never eaten the bread of the whiteman. They don't depend on the Bureau of Indian Affairs or anyone else. They live entirely on their own resources.

When they want food, they kill whatever is near—whiteman's cattle, deer, or donkey. They raise crops in the mountains. They have never come down and embraced this society.

"These brothers, when they heard of my work, gave me these coins. See the dates? They range from 1832 to 1891. I am certain they would be of value to collectors, but their real value lies in the fact that they are medicine coins. There are four of them. Four is a symbol of completeness to our society. Four is representative of medicine itself.

"One time a Flathead Indian I had befriended was left in charge of our place while I was gone. His loyalties were more to the firewater bottle than they were to the tribe. He couldn't really understand what we were doing in the Bear Tribe, even though we had taken him in and tried to help him. He stole my medicine coins and took them with him to Montana. My brother, Sun Dancer, who is also a Flathead, went up there and brought them back. The man understood that he must return them when he learned the coins were medicine."

What other medicine items do you carry?

Sun Bear: "I have in my own medicine bag a stone given to me by my sister Wabun. I have a meditation stone that comes from the Orient. Here is a shamrock that was given to me by one of the Irish who feels very strongly about his people. I have a piece of turquoise.

"The Bear Tribe has a medicine bundle with a pipe. There is a patch of cloth that has the blood of all our brothers and sisters on it. Whenever a person takes a blood oath to the Bear Tribe, his blood goes on that patch. Our bundle also has medicine stones in it. The pipe is of catlinite and it has feathers and things that people have given it."

Dallas Chief Eagle: "I have a rattle, a very special rattle. The Yuwipi people told me that if I should ever lose it, I would only have to go back to a certain place in South Dakota, and it would be there waiting for me. You will never see a rattle of this type in any museum. It is too sacred. One time I tried to get its beat on a tape, but it was impossible to record it. Whenever I go on any trips, I always carry my rattle with me."

What is the meaning of the pendant around your neck, Chief Eagle?

Dallas Chief Eagle: "It is the Indian star. The Star of David has six points; the Star of Bethlehem has five; and the Indian star has eight points. The colors of red, yellow, black, and white are sacred colors to the plains people, particularly the Cheyenne. There is no special medicine significance to the pendant, however."

How do you use your dreams to give you direction?

Sun Bear: "I use my dreams in many ways. I use them as a sense of warning to advise my brothers and sisters against danger. I use dreams to give me ideas to develop later. I have even used my dreams in gambling.

"Some things that I see, I cannot always tell my people, because they are not yet ready. I know of certain shortcuts to get to where we have to go. In medicine, some things are of value to yourself personally. Like some medicine people have power chants which can be passed down and used by only one family."

Twylah: "I follow very closely the goals which I have set for myself, so my personal symbols appear not only in my dreams, but in everything I do. One of my symbols is the circle. It is balance, equality, unity. To me, dreams are guidelines. And my dreams and visions come to me by day, as well as by night.

"But I do not force things. I do not go to bed with a problem on my mind and think that it will be solved by morning. I do not feel that I can force the dream, but what I can do is to open myself and become receptive. My advice to anyone is to open up and let the thing come down to you."

Do you think that dreams that might come through a chemical stimulus would be as reliable as dreams that come naturally?

Twylah: "I have never used anything of that sort, so I am not in a position to give feeling toward it. I cannot answer for anyone else. My opinion is that the dream or vision would not be as pure as that which came through a natural opening-up. I think that anything that would be forced would have its limitations."

What about the vision quest? How should one go about preparing for it?

Dallas Chief Eagle: "First, I would tell the seeker to cleanse himself spiritually. Take a sweat bath. After this, don't touch any food. You may drink some water. Go somewhere where you will have a minimum of interference. Then, sitting, kneeling, or standing, meditate. Think on why you are there.

"Between a day and a half to three days, I should say within four days, the message will come. The message may be received in English or in some other language, but you will understand it, the entire concept. Or you might receive the message in the form of a chant. In ancient times, Indians sang their prayers, because they felt singing was of a higher level than ordinary speech."

Sun Bear: "I did not go on my actual vision quest until I was in my twenties. Before the coming of my realization of what I must do with my life, I spent much time seeking my direction and learning from accomplished medicine people. I spent time with the Hopis, the Navajos, and many other tribes. I learned from the Peyote brothers, and I gained respect for their medicine. Since those days, medicine has come to me at different times and in different ways.

"One time I was on top of a mountain when I received a vision of an earthquake. The next day, I called a friend in Los Angeles, and things had happened as I had seen them in my vision.

"In other visions, I have seen the destruction of the system. I have seen armies and bands roaming the cities. I have seen bands made up of former policemen gathering up their brothers and fighting to stay alive against bands made up of revolutionaries who gathered when they saw this nation, this system, being broken down by natural disasters. When the Great Cleansing comes, there will be many who will pick at the bones of the dying system."

What techniques do you employ to stop the world, to enter deep states of meditation?

Dallas Chief Eagle: "I think the mind can be made to absorb itself and expand itself. I think one can do intense meditation, and I think one can cultivate this ability. I concentrate intensely on a subject. I assume no special body position. I take careful pains to guard against being disturbed. I've tried to meditate in forests and beside streams where there was too much interference. I must reach an area of complete solitude. If one gains a proper avenue for introspection, the mind absorbs itself—then explodes, bringing knowledge to the seeker.

"I think this knowledge comes from a higher power. Sometimes when you speak in this area, you lose a lot when you use the term 'God.' You may lose proper perspective of a subject that has become so associated in our society with Christianity that God is considered only from that point of view.

"I think there are levels of power and intelligence, and I believe you can reach a definite higher level of energy through meditation and intense concentration. I don't think it takes the mind long to grow accustomed to rising to higher levels and to learn how to gain proper knowledge from different levels of energy and power. I think it is quite possible to train the mind to reach these unknown dimensions."

Twylah: "I can get off the world very easily. One of my devices is to put myself in a mental drain tile. I put spiritual protection around everyone, and then I place it around myself so there is complete balance. All the spiritual forces are opened up so they can circulate and everything goes in balance.

"When one is in the process of learning, the material world can be so pronounced that the student leans in the direction of worldliness. The spiritual self does not come through because it is being shut off. In order for the spiritual light to function the way it should, the teacher has to do something drastic to make the student stop what he is doing wrong and get him back to the real thing—learning about himself and his environment.

"I'll tell you how I used to meditate with my grandfather, Moses Shongo. In the morning we would sit on the porch and watch the sun as it would come up. We would say thanks for the things for which we were grateful—things below the ground, on the ground, above the ground. In other words, we would progress from the material to the spiritual.

"The moment you are born, you breathe in the breath of life, the most important gift of the material world; but prior to birth, you have been endowed with the spiritual light. The spiritual light lives within the fetus. When you are born and you are dunked in the clear spring water to take your first breath, you receive the gift of life, which will help you in the world of material evolution.

"At the end of the day, we would go again to the front porch and watch the sun drop down behind the trees. Grandpa would say, 'It is time to deal with nature.' And we would open ourselves and pray. The prayers were always those of thanksgiving.

"In order to ensure solitude, one should practice visualizing a spiritual circle around himself. This process rekindles yourself and keeps an aura close around you. Everyone has an area around himself that is his own residence. Sometimes he will permit certain people he loves to enter this circle.

"The early Seneca meditated very often on how best to achieve self-improvement. He made an honest study of his personal self, both good and bad. He decided what changes he wanted to make in his personal self-pattern. He listed the personal habits he wished to establish, and he listed the personal habits he wished to break.

"One must always evaluate the goals which he is contemplating. Will your goals of self-improvement bring about an expansion of positive experiences?

"Examine your environment. Do you control your environment, or does it control you?

"Seek new dimensions of awareness by looking around you and discovering that which directly affects you.

"Tap into your creative ability and raise your highest intellectual self. Discover personal techniques whereby you might better control your gifts and abilities. Raise your perception to the unlimited level of spirituality.

"Your own personal symbolism can enable you to establish a focal point for meditation. If you believe that you need some kind of gimmick to aid in your self-development, don't go out and buy some tacky external thing. Discover a personal symbol that truly fits your own personality.

"The ancient Senecas taught their children to pray at an early age. The children would pretend that they were in council. They would pray in thanksgiving. This was their first introduction to going into the Silence, seeking self-development, and offering proper prayers.

"The young Seneca were told to tap into their highest intellectual awareness.

"They were told not to force awareness. This is a passive state that must come at its own pace.

"They were instructed that prayer was a creative process that began with an idea. Prayer must be accompanied with feeling. This is so important. You cannot have prayer without having a definite idea accompanied with feeling.

"They were taught that in order to have a prayer fulfilled, it is necessary to understand the levels of feeling. This understanding must exist before desires and actions can be controlled.

"One of the first things Seneca children learned was that they might create their own world, their own environment, by visualizing actions and desires in prayer. A child will create his own world through imagery. He will create his own environment. This is a natural gift with which we are all born. The Senecas believed that everything that made life important came from within. Prayer assisted in developing a guideline toward discipline and self-control.

"I am saddened by the fact that today's parents do not discipline their children on a very high spiritual level. This is so important, Brad."

Indeed it is, Twylah. This kind of discipline has to do with how to instill proper values, with how best to educate the young person to grow so that the parents might at the same time continue their own growth. Twylah, would you give us an example of a proper prayer, one that could be given in the correct attitude of thanksgiving, rather than that of supplication?

Twylah: "Yes, Brad, I would be happy to share one of my own:

O Great Spirit, I awake to another sun,
Grateful for gifts bestowed, granted one by one.
Grateful for the greatest gift, the precious breath of life.
Grateful for abilities to guide me day and night.
As I walk my chosen path of lessons I must learn,
Spiritual peace and happiness, rewards of life I learn.
Thank you for your spiritual strength, and for my thoughts to pray;
Thank you for your infinite love that guides me through the day.

Chief Eagle, Twylah has told us that she is often aware of the presence of her ancestor, the great chief Red Jacket. Although we have discussed your emulation of Crazy Horse's ideals, do you feel any identification with your ancestor?

Dallas Chief Eagle: "Yes, I do. I am descended from Crazy Horse on my mother's side. Crazy Horse was a mystic. He had the ability to go to another level of intelligence, another level of energy. He developed his mind very keenly. The Indians called him a quiet man, not a strange man, as has been so often said. The Sioux people understood these things.

"My grandfather had the ability to leave his shadow. Yes, that is what I said. The sun could be out bright, and he would just walk away from his shadow.

"Yes, that is illogical. Levitation is illogical. Reading peoples' thoughts is illogical. Many things that our people take for granted are considered illogical by the dominant society.

"Once when I was camping with my family in the mountains, my boy was climbing high on a teepee pole. A medicine person named Foggy Bird came over to visit me. Just then my little boy slid down the pole onto a bed of cactus. He was screaming in pain. I asked Foggy Bird to help me.

"He pulled down my boy's pants and yanked some of the needles out, but I know he didn't get them all. He spat on the boy's rump and said some prayers. Right then my boy went limp. I thought he had fainted, but Foggy Bird told me he was only sleeping.

"My boy was asleep for maybe an hour and a half when we got him up. He awoke without a mark on his rump. Just before Foggy Bird started spitting and praying, I saw actual large, white lumps where the needles were. After the boy's sleep, all traces of the terrible pricks had disappeared. To this day, my son knows nothing of what happened."

I believe that one of the basic essentials in medicine power is a belief in a total partnership with the world of spirits and the ability to make personal contact with grandfathers and grandmothers who have changed planes of existence. In today's society, many people would feel awkward about recognizing a partnership with the spirit world. What advice could you give to a person who might say "I can go along with vision quests, dream teachings, walking in balance on the Earth Mother, but once you are dead, you are dead. I want to follow medicine power, but I cannot accept a spirit world."

Twylah: "The first thing that I would say to such a person would be to ask him if he had ever had an experience that made him wonder if there might not be a possibility of a spirit world. If the person were reluctant to discuss this, I would ask him if he feared death. If he did and he admitted to this fear, I would ask him just what put the fear into him. Was it religious teachings? A dread of the unknown?

"In either case, I would say that fear has a great deal to do with his rejection of spirits. Immediately, the person rejected the notion of spirits on an intellectual level, but his judgment was influenced by an emotional level. When you confront the person with this, you must ask him to decide where he resides on an emotional level. Nine times out of ten, this tack opens a person up, because he must talk about this and look at it from another approach than the one with which he was familiar.

"Then I might ask if he has ever thought strongly of a loved one who has passed over. Had it ever occurred to him that he may have had that strong thought because the person was close to him in spirit at that moment? I would suggest that the next time he had this sensation that he have a conversation with the person in spirit. I can promise that he will have a wonderful feeling.

"Some people will open up right away and say, 'Yes, I did have such an experience.'

"For those who have never had such an experience, or will not admit to one, I can promise a wonderful feeling if they will try it the next time they have a strong thought of someone in spirit.

"You have to have a place to begin with people, and this very small, insignificant way can start the seed growing. Once a person opens up, the entities, the spirits, will come.

"Everyone wants proof of survival in spirit, and so did I. I have many times over proved the existence of the spirit world to my own satisfaction.

"Another thing, talking to others who have had experiences with spirits helps a person get over being embarrassed about such matters. If you are in a group and their vibrations are in harmony with yours, you can grow in spiritual matters and be supported by others.

"The most important thing in medicine is the importance of balancing the human being as he should be governed by the laws of nature. I don't think that to seek this balance is to turn back. If we turn toward our highest intellectual selves and begin to listen to our creative selves, we would certainly have more peace of mind.

"The Indian has always known that in order to keep his peace of mind, he must keep his balance with nature. He knew that the minute he became out of balance with nature, he was going to have trouble. The moment *anyone* is out of balance with nature, *he is in trouble!*

"Even if you live in a large city, you can still keep somewhat in balance with nature. You can know what foods are best for you. You can know how much sleep you need, and how you can best adjust to your individual cycles.

"Yes, I think that if a person truly wants to have a peaceful life in the midst of turmoil, he can have it. But he must learn to establish a balance and to control his own thoughts, so that he can look at the material world and see it for what it really is. That world of noise and confusion is for controlling, not for wallowing."

Dr. J.T. Garrett is a medicine practitioner uniquely qualified to comment upon the practical and modern aspects of the traditions of his people, the Cherokee. Currently the Health Systems Administrator for the Cherokee Indian Hospital in Cherokee, South Carolina, Dr. Garrett wrote to compliment me that my earlier works on medicine had constituted a "...dynamic representation of Indian beliefs and the revival of our spiritual heritage."

For this volume, I have invited Dr. Garrett to share his experiences with "Doc" Amoneeta Sequoyah, a Cherokee medicine man. According to Dr. Garrett:

"Amoneeta was willing for me to share certain aspects of Indian medicine. I know well the aspects not to be shared with others. Doc foresaw an increased interest in the traditional heritage and culture among Indians and certain non-Indians. Your work seemed to tap that source of interest with numerous Indian medicine people from various tribes. Amoneeta's response to your publication was, 'Yeah, that's right. He's got the right information from some good people who know about these things (Indian medicine).'

"The Cherokees continue to preserve their medicine traditions and to integrate many of those sacred ideas in our present health system. I am submitting the following in the hope that it will be used in respect of our sacred ways."

Indian Medicine—A New Era

"Traditional Indian medicine is very much alive to many Indians, and it is also a traditional myth for a few skeptics. The respect for this ancient medicine tradition is still held by Indian people, although few Indian people will discuss fully the impact of Indian medicine on tribes today. According to the medicine elders, we must retain the tradition and sacredness of the medicine ways or Indian people will fade into history.

"There is a fear in sharing Indian medicine ways, which is that sharing ancient traditions will result in loss of the last Indian resource. Therefore, there is a growing interest among Indian people in learning and preserving medicine traditions for the yet unborn.

"It seems unfortunate that our young Indians do not hear the stories of our traditions as they were once told. These stories shared a feeling along with a belief. They integrated life on the Earth Mother, as well as the life hereafter. More Indian people are realizing what has been lost with the passing of each elder. Indians and non-Indians alike are acutely aware of the need to talk and to listen to our elders. Maybe all has not been lost as a new era of Indian medicine emerges."

AN EMERGING SPIRIT

"The term 'spiritual' implies a religious native relating to a divine belief. Among Indians, the term 'spirit' implies a more active personal involvement with the supernatural, experiencing a quality or feeling with the Great Spirit. Many Indian people are awaiting the return of Indian spirit to Indians or the 'real people.' Some Indian prophets foresee the spirit emerging with trauma or with a special person.

"Brad Steiger has contributed to the revival of the Indian medicine heritage. Many Indian people speak openly of the emerging spirit. In *Warriors of the Rainbow,* William Willoya and Vinson Brown relate the prophetic dreams of Indian people. The visions mentioned by the prophets stressed the need to seek harmony with a revived purity of our minds.

"The interest of non-Indians and the rekindled interest of many Indians seem to reinforce the emerging spirit of Indian medicine. The purpose for sharing my thoughts and experiences is to relate the spirit of Indian medicine. This is taken from my apprenticeship with our traditional medicine man, 'Doc' Amoneeta Sequoyah. Our sharing was an opportunity for the traditional medicine ways to be integrated with the current approach to health and medicine. Ironically, modern health and medicine is realizing the concept of Indian medicine ways. These writings introduce a new medicine era. It started with the emerging spirit that is returning to Indian people."

MEDICINE OR HOLISTIC WAYS

"The holistic approach provides a renewed sense of direction for putting the humanistic aspect back into medicine. It still does not go as far as Indian medicine did toward including a person's involvement with his own health.

"Our modern physicians have assumed a tremendous responsibility for patients that seems unnecessary. Many physicians have taken away the power of choice and individual involvement in one's health, happiness, and well-being.

"Holistic medicine comes closer to including the personal dignity so desperately needed by all of us. Indian medicine ways were just that—ways for continued personal dignity in making individual choices about life and the life hereafter. Modern medicine is realizing the tremendous power of Indian medicine as an emerging spirit.

"Psychologists and psychiatrists today have managed to classify people to the point that frightens our old medicine men. The manipulative power of this classification system can destroy the spirit of human beings.

"At least most psychics still allow people to make choices about their future. The narrowed thinking of some psychologists can result in conditioned living taking away the unique spirit of a person. There are also some psychologists who have taken conditioned masses of people back to the realization of individual choices in quality of lifestyle.

"Indian medicine should have gotten proper credit for theories including the psychoanalytic ideas of Sigmund Freud, analytic thinking of Carl Jung, holistic or individual approaches of Alfred Adler, the psychology of consciousness of William James, the client-centered perspectives of Carl Rogers, and the Gestalt approach suggested by Frederick Perls.

"Indian medicine ways were sacred because they represented the traditions Indians followed for hundreds of years. These traditions affected tribal members as a way of life and life hereafter. The affect on an individual was an effect on the spirit of a person.

"There was nothing more respected and cherished than the spirit of a person. This was sacred because a person's spirit was like the Great Spirit. That dignity of a person must always be held sacred as Indian people have always believed. It is held sacred by respect and love for each self and all around the self.

"Therefore, Indian medicine ways go far beyond our current views on holistic medicine ways. These things were taught in an apprenticeship with an elder medicine man or shaman. Learning to control medicine power and how to use it to help people requires a relearning process. This process will be discussed while preserving the sacredness of medicine ways."

RELEARNING THE WAYS

"My apprenticeship in Indian medicine represented a renewal in teaching a preserved tradition. The medicine man is still a respected position among the eastern band of Cherokee Indians. This tribe continues to recognize the traditional council concept of group leadership. Council members are elected with a tribal chairman. The council acts as a legislative group working closely with the chief and his executive group, providing direction for all tribal members. There are over 8,000 tribal members on the Indian rolls recognized by the federal government on the boundary or reservation in western North Carolina.

"The medicine man has lost the civil recognition of earlier years. Therefore, the position of medicine man, while highly respected, has been reduced to a society position. This has proved valuable in keeping close to tribal members and in touch with the real needs of Indian people. According to our medicine elders, this was by design to preserve tradition and to retain sensitivity to the needs of Indian people.

" 'Doc' Amoneeta Sequoyah was our traditional medicine man. He was highly respected within the medicine circle of Indians all over America. There were some Indians and non-Indians who found it difficult to understand him. He was like a man placed one hundred years after his time to help people understand what they had lost. Doc Sequoyah passed on to the other world in August of 1981.

"Four years before his passing, he insisted that I learn the medicine ways and return to the reservation. Four years ago this was an impossible dream for me. As Doc Sequoyah has said, I returned over a year ago to administer our health and hospital program. According to his vision, traditional medicine ways are being integrated in our modern health setting.

"Doc Sequoyah said that my apprenticeship started with my grandfather. He worked with Amoneeta, as I prefer to call him, during the building of railroads and roads for travel and progress. As they saw this progress, they knew that people would change, and Indian medicine would be lost without forethought.

"My grandfather taught me to respect tradition and to maintain pure thought. He taught me to appreciate mother nature and to stay close to Mother Earth as nourishing to one's soul. He knew the power of Indian medicine. All this was to focus for me almost thirty years after his passing when Amoneeta said, 'Well, are you ready? You've wasted too much time already.' It started with relearning the medicine ways.

"There is so much misunderstanding about Indian medicine. This has lead to skepticism and undue criticism. The herbal formulas and their use are really just one aspect of Indian medicine. This facet is often treated as being synonymous with Indian medicine, even among some Indians. It should also be understood that each tribe of Indians has its own medicine ways with similarities and peculiarities unique to Indian people. There is a common language in Indian medicine. It would be nice if everyone understood more about Indian medicine and treated the subject with greater respect. As Amoneeta once said, 'You can't decide that [medicine ways] for people. They have to decide that for themselves.' "

INDIAN MEDICINE SPIRIT

"Amoneeta once said, 'The Spirit has to come back to our people. Some won't even know the difference, but people will feel the spirit.'

"I wondered how things would be different. He responded, 'It's not what you know; it's what you feel inside that makes a difference. Medicine [ways] will give our people a feeling of belonging again. They will come together in the circle, caring for each other, helping each other. But they gotta have some pain first. Indians sure have had that!'

"He helped me to feel pain and to experience the medicine spirit, sometimes called medicine power.

"There have been medicine apprentices who have gotten too involved in the power aspects or have 'gone into the darkening land,' as Amoneeta would say. Carlos Castenada experienced this feeling in his writings on Don Juan. Psychologists Carl Jung and William James wrote of this experience of 'going over' with the fears of not returning to life. These people also realized the difficulty that apprentices have in explaining their experiences to others. It is reasonable to understand why medicine men are careful in what they share.

"The spirit of Indian medicine is understood by some non-Indians who have developed a heightened sensitivity. The 1960s brought many of these persons to public view in discussions of psychics and persons who acutely understood Indian concerns. The medicine spirit is realized by persons who experience an elated and anxious feeling about themselves and helping others. Amoneeta understood this feeling while helping others to seek their vision.

"Unfortunately, many people assume that a vision is something that only a select few experience. Like many others, it took me a long time to learn how to get back in touch with myself enough to seek my vision. Awareness is a start toward seeking a vision and having the spirit emerge. Hopefully, my sharing will help others become aware of the tremendous power within all of us.

"As Amoneeta once said, 'I'm old now, and I've done some things. Now it is time for me to look at what's ahead of me. Now it is time for you to learn how to carry this [medicine] on so people can understand.'

"According to Amoneeta, 'Something is happening that I can't tell you about just now. You gotta believe some things as they are. It's kinda like having faith in something.'

"At that time, we were discussing health issues. Amoneeta was a man of simple education with a tremendous depth of understanding. He had almost eighty years of living knowledge when discussing this subject. He said, 'In my day you had to prove you had the know-how to help people. Now they just take some classes in school and show you a degree. We had to learn all we could cause we didn't have a book to look at. You see, you had to be an artist like the carpenters used to be. You [medicine men] were sensitive to how people felt about themselves. Now doctors treat you on how they feel.' He was explaining the spirit of Indian medicine as a sensitive tool developed by the medicine men to 'read' a person coming to them.

"Amoneeta said that heart disease, cancer, and arthritis did not exist among Indians before the non-Indian came to our shores. He said that Indian medicine had to change and is still changing to help people. It seemed ironic to me that our basic concerns about health were so similar even though our backgrounds were so different.

"Amoneeta explained that the medicine spirit was the same in both of us. He would say that Indian medicine is a 'calling' that certain persons would sense or their parents would sense at an early age. As he would say with his quiet humor, '[Indian] medicine is like a woman who chases you until you catch her. Maybe that's the reason our medicine has such strong (spirit) ways.' "

CIRCLE TEACHINGS

"The 'Circle Teachings' were referred to by Amoneeta Sequoyah as a way of getting around to the real truths. These teachings seem very similar to thoughts expressed by many psychologists. As an example, Frederick Perls expressed the idea that people create their own world in Gestalt psychology. Indian medicine teaches the spiral toward perfection that each of us must accept to follow medicine ways. Psychologist Alfred Adler created many thoughts about humanistic psychology, which is similar self-searching through a vision quest. Carl Jung identified the importance of introverted and extroverted types in thinking, feeling, sensation, and intuitive thought. The intuitive process was realized by Carl Jung as he skirted the spirit world. He must have come very close to touching the real self as a small planet in the spirit universe. William James understood medicine control, commonly referred to as biofeedback today. Medicine men learned physical, mental, and spiritual control. The 'Medicine Triangle' simplistically presents this concept. Medicine men taught this concept as a discipline.

"Two psychologists came very close to the Spirit of Medicine in their experience and writings. Carl Rogers realized the concept of real and ideal self in working with group dynamics. He also used a passive counseling therapy approach. Indian medicine taught these concepts and used the family in the healing process. The responsibility for the illness or condition like the self was never taken away from the person. Wilhelm Reich in his research with 'Orgone' or bioenergy realized the importance of tension-relaxation and deep breathing. Indian medicine focused these concepts in utilizing a sweat lodge, a cold plunge into water, and ceremonial dancing. Reich's *Psychology of the Body* came close to the medicine teachings of body discipline and endurance with the spirit of an individual.

"Many more concepts are taught in Indian medicine before an apprentice has fully learned medicine techniques. The bottom line is the Circle of Life. This represents the way these teachings are applied to living. It is this love of living, this love of fellow man that Indian medicine teaches.

"Indian medicine teaches that everything returns into the circle like the sun rising each day and setting each night. It also teaches that every circle must be completed in everything we do, so the sun can continue to rise. Our lives seem to need this same consistency or cycle. If that circle is left incomplete, there is stress or vibrational interference affecting the physical, mental, and spirit being. This represents a small segment of the 'circle teachings.' "

ANCIENT TRADITIONS

"The ancient traditions in Indian medicine of all tribes required strict discipline. Traditions varied while certain ancient rites were common.

As an example, ceremonies included sacred traditions that have common origins. Prayers or chants were to the creator(s). The sun seemed always important in these ceremonies. In ancient Cherokee rites, Father Sun was recognized for assisting Mother Earth in creating roots and herbs used for medicine. If the plants failed to cure, however, it was the moon's fault. Special homage was paid to the moon for favor. These were not considered duties. They were considered as paths to truths.

"Fire was an agent as herbs were agents. Many customs utilized fire. Smoke from special fires acted as a messenger conveying the prayer on high.

"The uses of certain minerals were important in ancient traditions. Such things are not taken lightly even today. A charm given is something treasured or handled cautiously.

"According to Amoneeta, 'You gotta learn to live in harmony with everything around you. You let the plants and animals know you mean good, and they'll be good to you. They can be your helpers [agents]. The old medicine men taught us this. When someone gives you something, it may just be a little stone, hold on to it.'

"It seems this ancient tradition is returning in the new era of medicine. Some of these charms were used in psychic activities. Amoneeta called these things 'tricks.' His uncanny ability to use psychometry and psychically move inanimate objects always fascinated. Such 'tricks' would amaze me. Amoneeta would say, 'That's no big thing. Anybody can learn [to do] that.'

"The tradition of sensing or 'reading' things and people is still taught in Indian medicine. My ability to utilize this natural ability always seemed lacking.

"There was an occasion when I was putting up a television antenna for Amoneeta outside of his trailer. It was about fifteen degrees outside, no wind, and snow covering the ground. We were trying to get *anything* on the television. All we could get was a snowy picture—inside and outside! We were set on watching a football game when a woman drove up to the trailer.

"Amoneeta's first reaction was, 'I don't know why she's come here, she's not going to listen anyway.'

"From a distance, she appeared nice looking and non-Indian. The visitor was rather obese, but lively. She quickly appeared at the doorway, bringing a cake and some commodity foods. After niceties, the woman was ready for some heavy conversation. I got the hint to finish putting up the antenna.

"After absorbing more heat from the wood stove, I went out into the snow—but I could still hear some of the conversation. She wanted to learn some medicine traditions. Being rather persistent she asked, 'How do I learn mind projection versus out-of-body experience?'

"I caught a glimpse of Amoneeta's side profile that reminded me of an old picture of an elder Indian. He appeared stern and wise. He caught my eye then turned to the woman and said, 'You see that boy [pointing to me] out there? I've been watching him, and he's not getting it right. Hey! [getting my attention] What did you call that thing that measures the picture?'

"I told him it was a field strength meter. He continued, 'Well, that's what you [the woman] need to do with your mind. That's like picking it up with your mind. [You] would learn something if [you would] listen.'

"Ancient traditions taught what is now referred to as 'wind projection.' It was fairly easy to learn. Out-of-body, or 'going on a journey' as Amoneeta referred to it, was learned only by a few medicine men.

"Amoneeta turned to the woman and said, 'All you have to do is put your mind on where it is you want to be and just go on a journey.' The woman looked perplexed. She continued to question him for some secret. The woman left shortly afterward. An ancient tradition was given to her, but did she hear it.

"I rushed inside after connecting the wire to the antenna. After warming up and having some coffee, the TV was turned on. Amoneeta smiled and chuckled as nothing was on the TV but snow.

"Amoneeta said, 'You didn't get the signal. Of course, you don't sometimes [he chuckled]. Why don't you try using what he gave you.' My puzzled look prompted him to say, 'Are you going to do like that woman or listen?'

"Something was telling me inside to go back out in the cold and check the antenna. I was surprised to find a terminal connection that had become loose from my twisting the antenna. My previous thoughts had been to move the mast or to twist the antenna more, but not to check the terminal connections.

"Amoneeta and I spent the remainder of the afternoon talking Indian medicine and watching the last half of the football game. As Amoneeta said, 'The ways of our grandfathers are not just given to you, you gotta learn them just like they did. We're too educated now to understand these things. We doubt everything too much. The old medicine men taught these things."

A NEW ERA

"In recent years many young people came to Amoneeta excited about life. They wanted to learn and to seek their vision.

"It was different when one was an apprentice. The elder medicine men understood they would lose power as their apprentices learned and earned a reputation. In my case, it was understood that my vision was to help bridge a gap between modern thinking and traditional ways. I also understood being of age with gray hair before 'having the power to do these things,' as Amoneeta would say.

"Our young people could benefit from understanding their anxiousness as internal seeking. They are aware and uninhibited about understanding such techniques as projection, phasing-in-and-out, disengagement, spirit protection, circle teachings, and other ideas taught by our elders in stories. Such tales related these things on levels of awareness and understanding that resulted in changing interpretation and application as a person spiraled toward perfection.

"Doc Sequoyah referred to himself as an intervener rather than as a healer. In a sense, that seems to be what healing is all about. He never took credit for healing; he would let the person do that. I saw him as an artist more than a scientist.

"The new era of Indian medicine will continue to be ancient and traditional to Indian people. It will be an integration of modalities for non-Indian people with renewed possibilities for improving on our involvement in health maintenance.

"It may be best just to develop a new era, rather than comparing and analyzing, which Indian people do not need for acceptance. The negative impact of null testing is not acceptable to Indian people, because the element of faith as confidence is a measure of success rather than a result of success or failure. Our non-Indian physicians and health professionals are now beginning to learn about personal liability through malpractice. Maybe elder medicine men knew what they were doing when they would not work with non-Indians. Maybe all of us in the health field will eventually change our titles to health interveners.

"The future of Indian medicine is emerging from a past spirit for health action. Its focus will be on quality of life and planning for the life hereafter. As Doc Sequoyah once said, 'We have to believe that the Spirit of our Indian people is coming back. We have to believe that!' "

14
Walk in Balance

> O Great Spirit, bring to our white brothers the wisdom of Nature and the knowledge that if her laws are obeyed this land will again flourish and grasses and trees will grow as before. Guide those that through their councils seek to spread the wisdom of their leaders to all people. Heal the raw wounds in the earth and restore to our soil the richness which strengthens men's bodies and makes them wise in their councils. Bring to all the knowledge that great cities live only through the bounty of the good earth beyond their paved streets and towers of stone and steel.
>
> —Jasper Saunkeah, Cherokee

It was from Chippewa medicine man Sun Bear that I first heard the expression "Walk in Balance." That brief prayer-admonition presents the crux, the essence, and the ideal, of not only American Indian medicine power, but of all positive metaphysical doctrines.

Regrettably, Sun Bear, not everyone can go out into the hills and go to the mountaintop. Is it possible to walk in balance, to practice the ideals of Native American medicine if one lives in the concrete canyons of some large city?

Sun Bear: "You can practice medicine in the city or in any other place. I strive to practice it right here. Sometimes, you know, I have to stand aside for a while and just keep within my heart what I believe. A lot of people still can't comprehend medicine, but I don't put it out of my mind or out of my life just because there are people who are not yet capable of understanding it."

Some of the traditionalists have told me that they have to get back to Pine Ridge, to the Black Hills, to the mountains before medicine will work most effectively.

Sun Bear: "This is true within the hearts of many of those people. Right now I am working—between work on *Many Smokes* magazine and other things—to find ways to help keep some of my Indian brothers and sisters on the reservations so they don't have to come to the city and pay a hundred and fifty dollars a month rent, utilities, and the rest of it. I am trying to work it out so that by marketing their arts and crafts and other items, they might earn a hundred dollars extra to supplement their income and allow them to continue to live comfortably where they are."

You would agree with me that the psycho-religious system of the Native American may offer relevant spiritual guidance and a workable structure of applied metaphysics for us today?

Sun Bear: "I would agree with you. I think we offer a pattern of balance. We may not have all the answers that pat. Or maybe we have *all* the answers, but we don't have them in a manner that can be interpreted in a manner to be everything for everybody.

"You know, I accept a lot of the teachings of Gandhi. I think he was a great man. I find a lot of harmony with what he taught. I find no disharmony with the teachings of the carpenter of Nazareth, either. But I mean the *real* things he spoke of."

Christianity, then, not Churchianity.

Sun Bear: "Yes, I find that some of the double-mouthed people who go around claiming to rep for him and who put their blessings on the various military regimes of whatever country they inhabit are not my species of man."

But you do feel that medicine power can be used in any environment?

Sun Bear: "Yes. I have to deal with the world every day. I don't feel that I have to retreat into a cave with my rattle like some of my people want me to do. I don't feel that I have to be the kind of holy man who gets out of contact with the world. I feel that a good portion of my medicine is a battle with the world as it is now, trying to rectify, trying to build things that are beneficial both for my Indian people and my non-Indian people."

I personally applaud such a position. I have always felt that the holy man must be with the people, struggling with contemporary society as it exists, not sitting somewhere as a recluse, contemplating his navel.

Sun Bear: "Yes, I have used that same 'contemplating the navel' reference. Maybe I quote it too often, because I don't feel that just crying

'OM' and so forth is the total sum of humanity. If you aren't in the battle with life, doing something worthwhile for humanity, then it just isn't there. Cesar Chavez is a holy man in his way.

"The other thing of it is that you have to watch so that you don't misuse power. I have known both Indian and non-Indian leaders who have used power as a whip to take things for their own gain. Power is something you have to watch. You must maintain a balance.

"I try to ingrain in the Bear Tribe that we don't have to be a breechcloth-dragging outfit. Eating regularly is not immoral, either. One of my very close associates wanted me to set up a hierarchy, where nobody could talk to me except by special interview and so forth, but I couldn't see that."

I think we have enough hierarchies, secret societies, and exclusivities as it is.

Sun Bear: "Everyone must learn to walk with a good balance. They must learn that I can't just give them a daily transfusion of medicine power. This has been the problem of a lot of people who come to us saying they don't want the Establishment anymore, but they don't have the ability to balance themselves yet. This is where the big struggle is. It is a hard thing for the man who has not yet learned to carry the law within himself and to walk as a brother."

This is a hard thing. It is a contest for which one must constantly train. One must stay in good spiritual condition, as well as good physical condition. We have never been told it is going to be easy.

Sun Bear: "My medicine is for every day. It is not a thing for a Sunday treatment. Sometimes the Nez Perce or the Klamath or some other tribe call on me to come up. If my knowledge of economic development or how to create something will be satisfying to them on that level, I am happy to make it that way. I am capable of surviving successfully on that level. Because I have these talents, some people think that I am a promoter and so forth. But I can also take my jackknife out and skin three deer, or I can hoe a couple of acres of corn, if I have to. That is all part of the thing of it.

"The sad thing about this society is the fact that they have tried to put everything into little boxes. Religion is in this box, and religion doesn't have anything to do with the growing of corn or the making of love or anything else in those boxes over there. All things can come together in harmony. This is a natural thing, a balance thing. You can be a natural human being, blending in with the balance of everything, and you can be a medicine person, too.

"There are a lot of medicine men on the reservations across the country whose work is more with the herbs and with healing. There are different degrees of medicine men. Some work with healing and some work with things of a higher nature, where they call in spirit powers to work with them.

"They say that knowledge is also healing. If I can take my medicine and use my knowledge to heal the heads of people who are screwed up and going in six different directions . . . if I can bring a balance to them so that they can walk with a good balance on the Earth Mother, well, that is medicine and that is where the medicine power lies at this time—in teaching.

"If I wanted to go up and spend a month by myself on top of a mountain, I could perhaps generate the power to do some of the things our ancient medicine men did, like teleporting myself or like raising the lodge. This is real power, and it is something that a person can get if he really needs it. Maybe that is the medicine that will be there for me; maybe that is a part of it, but to me, the doing, the teaching, the helping is where my medicine is right now.

"Some of the things I must do are just dull, everyday things. We must figure out how to get better distribution for our books and our magazine, *Many Smokes.* We feel this is good knowledge, and it should be getting out to more people. We must plan how to move our people out on the land where we may have a permanent land basis. This is all part of living."

You may not be of the world, but you are in it, and you are going to have to survive.

Sun Bear: "Right. And it is a good thing. I don't feel restless or agitated, like a lot of other people feel, because they don't have their goals of tomorrow yet today. I feel content in what I am doing. I feel happy."

Don Wanatee is rather dubious about one's ability to practice medicine effectively while living in a large city.

Don Wanatee: "I feel that you have to go back to where the 'action' is, as they say. I don't think medicine can be practiced as effectively in the cities. I think that many of these Indians have lost their medicine, their religion, and they are trying to find another way to get it back. I would say that their journey, their search, is going to be difficult. I say that they must go back to their religious men to be taught, then they might have a chance."

Is it possible to rediscover *medicine power?*

Wanatee: "I think in so far as the Indian tribes are concerned, they have been given a way of life, a religion, a belief, a philosophy, or whatever it is; and if they have lost it, then certainly they will have some difficulty getting it back. If they are shown the way by somebody who has fasted and found the path again, I think they can revive it. But as far as white people are concerned, I think they are going to have to do more than just look. They are going to have to exert themselves, not only in the Indian ways, but in their own ways, whatever they may be. Their beliefs will have to be engraved right into their souls.

"Most whites believe in some form of Christianity. I hear that the 'freaks' [hippies] know the presence of a single God, but they are looking for a means of communication. The Mesquakies have no problem with communication. They have a direct line. They can still do the same things they did three or four hundred years ago.

"Some pockets of native belief are still present among the Sioux, but there are a great many areas where they have been converted to some other religion. The Sioux who want to go back to the old traditions have a far better chance of re-creating that religion than do the whites, who wish to acquire this tradition for the first time.

"I think that if the whites went back to the type of religion that was first given to them and really practiced it, they would be happier. Indian traditions and non-Indian traditions are not incompatible; but at the present time, I don't think they can really come together. We have maintained our beliefs and they are sacred to us. They demand an intense participation that becomes life itself, a total thing."

Rarihokwats, editor of *Akwesasne Notes,* recognizes that people other than Native Americans may develop a natural lifestyle and strive to live in total harmony with the Earth Mother and with the cosmos, but he issues certain cautions:

> The way too many people approach Christianity is to learn a certain number of formulas and rituals, believing that in the words there is some magic. What they don't understand is that those rituals and those words merge and become manifestations of certain feelings and certain attitudes, and that one who recites the Lord's Prayer or something without these feelings and attitudes really isn't achieving anything at all.
>
> There have been a lot of anthropologists who have criticized Indian medicine practitioners today by saying that their words are not accurate. They say they have a recording that was done in 1902 and

that the practitioner has changed the words and the ritual isn't correct. Well, of course, the practitioners have changed the words. The feelings and attitudes are the important ingredients.

I think that what is essential for those non-Indian people who are wanting to get something out of medicine power and find something in there for their own lives is that they make sure that they get this not by imitating and copying the Indian, but by developing their medicine in the same way that Indian people have developed this power.

Go to the waters and listen. Try to hear what it is that the waters have to say. What is the essence of the spirit of the waters?

The only formula is to go and sit and listen. This is what the non-Indian should do, rather than trying to take over what has already been developed by the Indians, because I don't think the non-Indian can do it.

On the other hand, we also recognize in other people who are living a natural life-style and who are living in harmony with all things, a high degree of brotherhood and unity. We recognize those people for who they are. I don't think they need to become Indians in the stereotyped meaning of that word. I think that where many people make their mistake is that they are trying to take on an Indian identity, rather than becoming a real person.

I would hope that people would just seek to become real people, whoever they are, and not attempt to be Indian.

I asked Dr. Walter Houston Clark if he considered it a step backward, intellectually and spiritually, to embrace a tradition that was in this continent before the whiteman came:

I think that the Indians have enormous contributions in their religious traditions and in their attitude toward the environment to make to the kind of dried-up, desiccated sort of civilizaton that typical America represents. I don't think we can turn back the clock to two or three hundred years ago, when there were great spaces all over the continent, but I do believe that in our metaphysics we have much to learn from the Indians.

At the same time, I think that the Indians have a great deal to learn from us. But we must start on a basis of mutual trust, mutual understanding. Profound mystical experiences have been shared between the whites and the Indians. I think that Carlos Castaneda's book *A Separate Reality* is a kind of indication of a community of interest and values at a very profound level. The separate reality of Don Juan is very similar to the enlightenment of Plato, when he uses his Allegory of the Cave. I think the essential message here is really the same, and here is just one example of a compatibility of a Western philosopher, who lived in another country and at a different age, with Don Juan, an Amerindian sorcerer. The essential

> beliefs and values are very similar, if not identical. It is at this level that I think there is a possibility that oil and water may mix. I hope that the Indians keep themselves at this level, then persuade the white people to meet them in this same area.
>
> About a year ago, I came across a statement from William James in which he says, 'The mother sea and fountainhead of all religions lie in the mystical experiences of the individual. All theologies, all ecclesiasticisms are secondary growths, super-imposed.' I seem to see an enlightenment coming into our young people so that those who come into contact with the Indian culture will find a much readier empathy and understanding than the typical orthodox churchgoer or church leader could ever understand.

For many years now, my own personal metaphysics have incorporated American Indian medicine.

I agree with William James's statement that the very essence of all religions lies in the mystical experiences of the individual, and I agree with Rarihokwats, who has told us that we should not imitate the American Indian's spiritual achievements, but that we should develop our own medicine in the same ways that the Indian developed medicine power—by going into the silence and listening. I also seek always to follow Sun Bear's admonition to walk in balance, to remain the spiritual warrior, struggling with contemporary society as it exists, devoting my strength to a disciplined and lifelong vision quest for knowledge.

I offer the following as examples of procedures employed in my personal medicine. They are not to be construed as guidelines, for, if pressed for advice, I will only echo the words of Rarihokwats: "The only formula is to go and sit and listen."

It is imperative in Native American medicine or in any practice of metaphysics to set a time apart to enable one to enter the silence. In my own practice, I have a daily exercise routine in which I work vigorously with barbells and dumbbells and ride a stationary bicycle in order to exert my physical body and distract my conscious self. I find that, just as one on a vision quest may deplete the physical self with monotonous and strenuous tasks in order to free the subconscious, so, for me, a workout with weights accomplishes this same goal.

After my period of purgative exercise, I enter a hot shower—in one sense, I suppose, the counterpart of the sweat lodge. After I have toweled dry, I lie flat on my back in a quiet place, apart from everyone and all distractions, and permit whatever is to come to me from the silence easy access to my heightened state of awareness.

For an added physical stimulus, I might wrap myself in a blanket, even covering my head. Such a withdrawal and sealing off increases the sensation of being totally isolated and permits one to become even less aware of the physical body and surrounding environment.

One may also smoke as an aid to meditation. The American Indian smoked by way of religious observance, not for personal pleasure. I recommend such a moderate usage of tobacco. Again, as a physical stimulus, offer the pipe (cigarettes or cigars are less preferable) to the four directions, upward to the Great Spirit, downward to the Earth Mother.

The puffs of smoke being carried toward the ceiling, or the sky, should represent one's thoughts, or prayers, being wafted to the Great Spirit. One should use these rhythmically released clouds of smoke as focal points for concentration. If one has achieved an attitude of calm before smoking, thoughts and images will begin to come almost at once. If one wishes, *Kinnikinnick* (Indian bark for smoking) can be obtained and used straight or mixed with tobacco in a pipe.

Traditional Native Americans carry a medicine bag that is filled with objects regarded as personally sacred to the bearer. The medicine bag can include objects symbolic of the four elements—fire, water, air, and earth. For example: a bit of obsidian, representative of fiery lava, or a bit of flint, the stone used to strike a fire; a small earthen water bowl or a dried water plant; a talon or feather from a bird; an unusual stone that for some reason caught the eye on a walk. One should remember that these objects, and any other items that may have personal significance to the bearer, serve as physical stimuli upon which the bearer might meditate in order to open the channel of the subconscious.

I believe that my dreams are telling me something about myself that I do not already know or that they are revealing patterns—future or present—of which it would be to my advantage to be made aware. Dream control is difficult, though hardly impossible, to learn, but anyone can keep dream diaries and maintain a permanent record of nightly assistance given by the unconscious—or, if you will, by the Great Spirit. Dream symbols are personal, and, while there seem to be universal images which bear consistently similar messages to dreamers in several cultures, one must come to self-knowledge during the vision quest in order to sort out glimpses of the future from bits and pieces of psychological garbage that are being vented by other levels of consciousness.

One may acquire a personal song or a mantra which facilitates meditation. Again, these songs are often given in dreams or in visions. Do not overlook certain pieces of music which contain personally nostalgic triggers. From time to time, I may employ a record of a song that is loaded with sentimental images for me. I find that the melody immediately sends me back to that particular experience; but after that moment in time has been relived, my unconscious is soaring here and there and often returning with valuable insights.

Do not neglect the Navajo Yeibichai or other recordings of Native American music. Recent New Age recordings would include, *Medicine Wheel: Music of the Metis.* Tom Bee's contemporary blend of tradition and rock can also inspire the seeker on his or her quest. A contemporary composer-artist I find particularly effective in assisting me to transcend the ordinary is Steven Halpern.

In our modern American society, one may become rather uneasy in stating a belief in a total partnership with the world of spirits, especially when we have learned so much about the limitless reach of the human psyche. One might begin by at least keeping the door open to the possibility that one may establish contact with those who have graduated to other planes of existence. With a small group of like-minded friends, one may begin to sit in development circles, remaining receptive to whatever communication might be channeled to any one of the circle. Under no circumstances should the situation be forced. A relaxed and tranquil state of mind will best permit the psyche to soar free of time and space and return with images, impressions, messages, and perhaps even an accompanying guide or a concerned entity. Each session should begin with each member of the circle asking a prayer for guidance and protection.

It is extremely difficult for those who live in contemporary society to "stop the world" and develop a "magic" or spiral time sense. Meditation affords the most effective method I know for allowing one to break free of the boundaries of conventional time. For a level of the unconscious, linear time does not exist. All is an eternal now. By utilizing any one of the meditative techniques discussed above, an altered state of consciousness may be achieved which will permit the meditator to enter that time-free, uncharted, measureless kingdom of the psyche.

We must learn to really see and to appreciate the adornments and trappings of the lovely Earth Mother. We must come to know that we are a part of the universe and that the universe is a part of us. We must recognize that the essence of the Great Spirit is to be found in all things, and all things are linked in ways that are as yet too subtle for our comprehension. We must bear our responsibility toward all plant and animal life with dignity, not with condescension.

In my opinion, a total commitment to such medicine power is in complete harmony with the basic tenets of all schools of positive metaphysical teachings and should be considered complementary to those bodies of philosophical thought which consider themselves to be orthodox religions.

Although I have long since abandoned anthropomorphic concepts of a Supreme Being, in moments of intense prayer I find myself speaking to the Great Spirit as if I were truly His/Her child. Intellectually, I know the truth of the relationship must be something very different and that to speak to All That Is as a parent is but a psychological device that is based upon my affection for childhood's image of my own parents, but the unconscious mechanism that is established enables us, I believe, to have an emotional sense of devotion and humility which will permit us to achieve the proper psychic attunement with that Supreme Intelligence that exists beyond our conscious self. If we have attained the proper spiritual linkup and not simply rattled off a prayer as if it were a religious nursery rhyme, we can come to feel in touch with an energy source outside of ourselves and we will come to feel a new power within our own being.

With thanks to my friend Iron Eyes Cody, here is a prayer that may be used by all who seek to walk in balance:

> Great Spirit, whose voice I hear in the winds and whose breath gives life to the whole world, hearken!
> I come before you as one of your many children. See, I am small and weak; I need your strength and wisdom.
> Permit me to walk in beauty. May my heart treat with respect the things which you have created; may my ears hear your voice!
> Make me wise that I may understand the things which you have taught, which you have hidden in every leaf and rock.
> I long for strength, not in order that I may overcome my brother, but to fight my greatest enemy, myself.
> Make me ever ready to come to you with pure hands and straight eyes, so that my spirit, when life disappears like the setting sun, may stand unashamed before you.

Brad Steiger

Brad Steiger, an internationally known psychic researcher, has authored more than 80 books in the metaphysical, psychic and inspirational fields. The motion picture rights for two of his books, *The Chindi* and *The Hypnotist,* have recently been sold. Steiger was also a writer of *Unknown Powers,* a 1978 film that won the Film Advisory Board's Award of Excellence. Some of his other works include *Brad Steiger Predicts the Future, True Ghost Stories, Astral Projection, Monsters Among Us, Mysteries of Time and Space, Atlantis Rising* and *The Star People* series. He and his wife Francie, a well-known psychic, live in Scottsdale, Arizona.

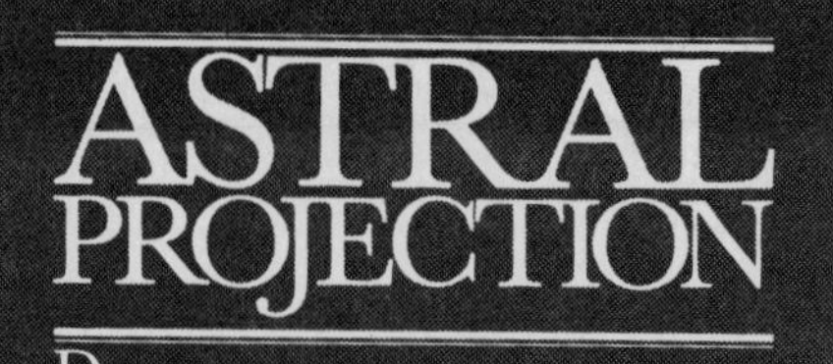

ASTRAL PROJECTION

by Brad Steiger

Parapsychological researchers have established that one of every one hundred persons has experienced out-of-body projection (OBE). These experiences are not limited to any single type of person, but rather they cross all typical boundaries.

In *Astral Projection*, Brad Steiger investigates the phenomenon of OBE and correlates those events into broad categories for analysis and explanation. In his clear and non-sensational style, Steiger relates how these spontaneous experiences occur and when they are likely to re-occur. In addition to the standard and well-documented categories of spontaneous astral projection at times of stress, sleep, death and near-death, Steiger devotes considerable time to the growing evidence for conscious out-of-body experiences, where the subject deliberately seeks to cast his or her spirit out of the physical shell.

Along with his study of astral projection, Steiger sets guidelines for astral travellers, tells them the dangers they may face and how this type of psychic experience might be used for medical diagnosis, therapy and self-knowledge.

Author Brad Steiger is your guide to controlling astral projection and using it for your own benefit.

ISBN 0-914918-36-2
234 pages, 6½" x 9¼", paper $12.95

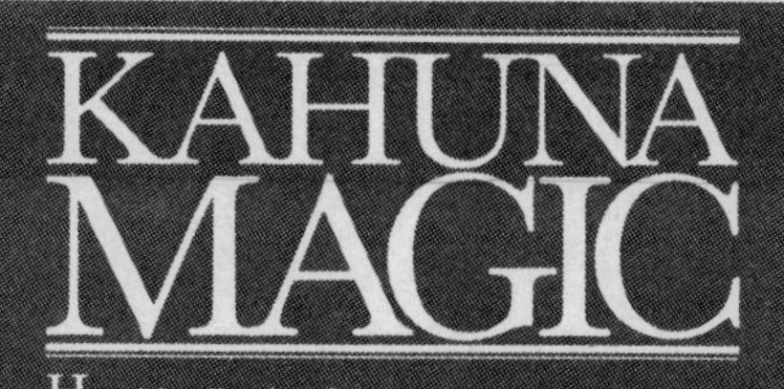

How Max Freedom Long rediscovered an ancient Hawaiian religion that delivers new insights into your hidden powers. Learn of your low self's innate control, how your middle self can receive telepathic messages and how your high self can change the future.

Brad Steiger

KAHUNA MAGIC

Brad Steiger

Based on the life work of Max Freedom Long, *Kahuna Magic* lays open the secrets of the Kahuna, the ancient Hawaiian priests. Long used the secrets of the Hawaiian language to unlock the secrets of this powerful and mystical discipline.

Long was a much-respected psychic researcher. His student Brad Steiger chronicles Long's adventures on the way to understanding the magic of the Kahuna. By following Long's trek, the reader will learn how the Kahunas used their magic for both the benefit of their friends and the destruction of their enemies.

Central to the Huna beliefs was the thesis that each person has three selves. The Low Self is the emotive spirit, dealing in basic wants and needs. The Middle Self is the self operating at the everyday level. The High Self is the spiritual being that is in contact with every other High Self.

The subject matter of *Kahuna Magic* is contemporary and compelling. The book incorporates many of the concepts and concerns of the modern Western psychological tradition of Jung and Freud while bringing in subjects as diverse as Eastern philosophies and yoga in a manner that will help the readers understand themselves and those around them.

ISBN 0-914918-34-6
127 pages, 6½″ × 9¼″, paper $10.95

TRUE GHOST STORIES

A Psychic Researcher's Hunt for Evidence of Hauntings

Brad Steiger

Brad Steiger's years of research into the infinite expanse of the spirit world is now available in this fascinating compilation of verified hauntings. These are not only the classic ghostly manifestations often discussed in paranormal literature, but also cases Steiger has researched, often using well-known mediums as contact points with the ethereal energies. *True Ghost Stories* does not stop at just relating the details of ghostly hauntings, it goes beyond other books on ghosts and hauntings to present the prevailing hypotheses about spirits in a scientific, yet highly readable manner.

The author investigates and explains three predominant theories that claim such manifestations are "telepathic infection," "idea patterns" or "psychic ether." Steiger concludes that no single one of these theories should be held dominant, but then again, none should exclude the other. *True Ghost Stories* proves the existence of ghosts and reveals significant facts and features of their nature. This new book leaves the reader with the chilling realization that we have yet to fully understand ghosts; more can be learned only through future contacts with the spirits.

ISBN 0-914918-35-4
220 pages, 6½" x 9¼", paper

$7.95

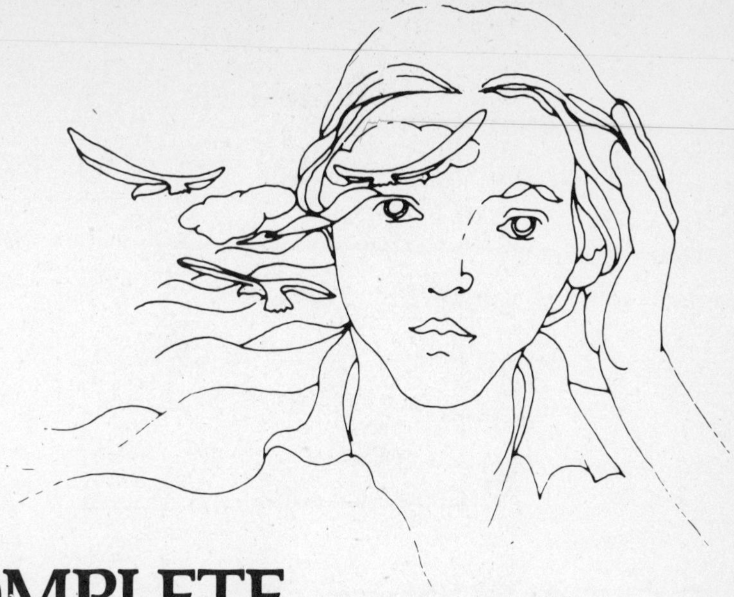

COMPLETE MEDITATION

Steve Kravette

Complete Meditation presents a broad range of metaphysical concepts and meditation techniques in the same direct, easy-to-assimilate style of the author's best-selling *Complete Relaxation*. Personal experience is the teacher and this unique book is your guide. The free, poetic format leads you through a series of exercises that build on each other, starting with breathing patterns, visualization exercises and a growing confidence that meditation is easy and pleasurable. Graceful illustrations flow along with the text.

Complete Meditation is for readers at all levels of experience. It makes advanced metaphysics and esoteric practices accessible without years of study of the literature, attachment to gurus or initiation into secret societies. Everyone can meditate, everyone is psychic, and with only a little attention everyone can bring oneself and one's circumstances into harmony.

Experienced meditators will appreciate the more advanced techniques, including more sophisticated breathing patterns, astral travel, past-life regression, and much more. All readers will appreciate being shown how ordinarily "boring" experiences are really illuminating gateways into the complete meditation experience. Whether you do all the exercises or not, just reading this book is a pleasure.

Complete meditation can happen anywhere, any time, in thousands of different ways. A candle flame, a daydream, music, sex, a glint of light on your ring. In virtually any circumstances. *Complete Meditation* shows you how.

ISBN 0-914918-28-1
309 pages, 6½" x 9¼", paper, $12.95

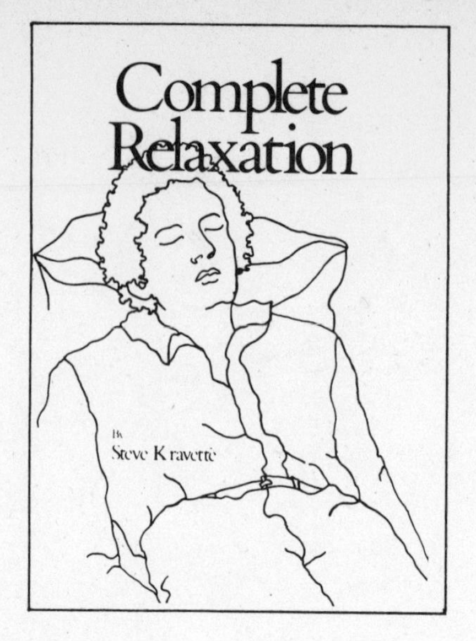

COMPLETE RELAXATION

Steve Kravette

Complete Relaxation is unique in its field because, unlike most relaxation books, it takes a completely relaxed approach to its subject. You will find a series of poetic explorations interspersed with text and beautifully drawn illustrations designed to put you in closer touch with yourself and the people around you. *Complete Relaxation* is written for all of you: your body, your mind, your emotions, your spirituality, your sexuality—the whole person you are and are meant to be.

As you read this book, you will begin to feel yourself entering a way of life more completely relaxed than you ever thought possible. Reviewer Ben Reuven stated in the *Los Angeles Times*, "*Complete Relaxation* came along at just the right time—I read it, tried it; it works."

Some of the many areas that the author touches upon are: becoming aware, instant relaxation, stretching, hatha yoga, Arica, bioenergetics, Tai chi, dancing, and the Relaxation Reflex.

Mantras, meditating, emotional relaxation, holding back and letting go, learning to accept yourself, business relaxation, driving relaxation.

Family relaxation, nutritional relaxation, spiritual relaxation, sensual relaxation, massage and sexual relaxation. *Complete Relaxation* is a book the world has been tensely, nervously, anxiously waiting for. Here it is. Read it and relax.

ISBN 0-914918-14-1
310 pages, 6½" x 9¼", paper

$10.95